LAPAROSCOPIC INGUINAL HERNIA REPAIR

Edited by

Ara Darzi MD FRCSI

John RT Monson MD FRCSI FRCS FACS

Illustrated by Dee McLean

I S I S
MEDICAL
MEDIA

Oxford

The Editors have asserted their right under the Copyright, Designs and
Patents Act, 1988, to be identified as the Editors of this work.

British Library Cataloguing in Publication Data.
A catalogue record for this title is available from the British Library

ISBN 1 8 99066 01 2

Library of Congress
Cataloguing-in-Publication Data

Darzi, A (Ara)
Laparoscopic Inguinal Hernia Repair/
Ara Darzi and John Monson

Always refer to the manufacturer's Prescribing Information before
prescribing drugs cited in this book.

Typeset by
Marksbury Typesetting Limited, Midsomer Norton, Bath, Avon

Printed and bound by
Dah Hua Printing Press Co., Ltd, Hong Kong

Distributors
Plymbridge Distributors Ltd, Estover PL6 7PZ, England

Contents

List of Contributors

William A. Brough BSc, MB, BS, FRCS
Consultant Surgeon, Stepping Hill Hospital, Stockport, UK

Albert K. Chin M.S.M.E., M.D.
Vice President of Research, Origin Medsystems Inc., Menlo Park, California, USA

James E. Coleman, MB, BSc(Hons), MS, MCh, FRCSI
*Honorary Consultant, Central Middlesex Hospital, London, UK
and European Medical Director, David & Geck/B Braun Dexon, Richmond,
Surrey TW9 1PJ, UK*

Ara Darzi MD, FRCSI
*Consultant Surgeon in Minimally Invasive Therapy
Department of Surgery, Central Middlesex Hospital, London, UK*

Arnold D.K. Hill M.Med Sci (Anat), FRCSI
Registrar in Surgery, Department of Surgery, Central Middlesex Hospital, London, UK

Austin L. Leahy MCh, FRCS, FRCSI
*Senior Lecturer in Surgery, Royal College of Surgeons in Ireland, Beaumont Hospital,
Dublin, Ireland*

Milton B. McColl MD
Vice President and Medical Director, Gynecare Inc., Menlo Park, California, USA

Frederic H. Moll MD
Vice President and Medical Director, Origin Medsystems Inc., Menlo Park, California, USA

John R.T. Monson MD, FRCSI, FRCS, FACS
*Professor of Surgery and Head of Department, University of Hull, Academic Surgical Unit,
Castle Hill Hospital, Humberside, UK*

Charles C. Nduka BA (Oxon) MB BS (Hons)
Surgical Houseman, Central Middlesex Hospital, London, UK

Henry Osborne MD FRCSI
Consultant Surgeon, Beaumont Hospital, Dublin, Ireland

Paraskevas A. Paraskeva BSc(Hons) MB BS (Hons)
Surgical Houseman, Central Middlesex Hospital, Park Road, London, UK

Akhtar D. Qureshi BSc, FRCSI, FRCS
Surgical Registrar, Castle Hill Hospital, Cottingham, Humberside, UK

Christopher M.S. Royston MB BS FRCS
Consultant Surgeon, Hull Royal Infirmary, Hull, North Humberside, UK

Allan D. Spigelman MB, BS, FRACS
Senior Lecturer and Honorary Consultant Surgeon, St Mary's Hospital Medical School,
Imperial College of Science, Technology and Medicine, London, UK

Preface

The development of minimal access surgery has probably been the biggest revolution in surgical practice in the last two decades. In many instances old operations such as cholecystectomy or fundoplication are simply being performed via a new route. In other cases however, new operations or approaches have been devised to address old problems. One such example of this is the repair of inguinal hernia. A not very glamorous operation has become the battlefield for opposing surgical opinion once again. Any brief review of the history of surgical repair of inguinal hernia will soon reveal that there are literally dozens of different operations – a sure sign that there is no clear answer available. The development of the laparoscopic approach is historically no different. Initially starting with simple closure of the deep ring with or without prosthetic plugs, tremendous hype was generated for this new approach. Fairly soon however, a more critical appraisal of the early results did not make pleasant reading, with high recurrence rates evident within one year of surgery. This realisation has lead to a more structured approach, with the development of automatically valid operations based on the knowledge gained from open surgery. However, the arguments still rage as fiercely as ever with laparoscopic enthusiasts claiming excellent results with patients returning to normal activity almost immediately following surgery. In contrast, the opposing view points to the disturbing accounts of new complications such as small bowel obstruction was sufficient reason to think again.

Of course the gold standard for hernia repair is pretty successful. Therefore the laparoscopic surgeons will have to provide convincing evidence that the new approach maintains the basic tenets of good surgery – safe, simple, cheap and effective – whilst developing the advantages of the minimal access route – less pain and improved cosmesis. This text does not attempt to provide the definitive answer to many of the questions. Rather we have taken a snapshot of the current techniques available – both open and laparoscopic – and have left it to the reader to decide the approach they wish to take. We have tried to present a balanced view, although individual contributors have been left to make their case as forcibly as they might see fit. Chapters on all the commonly employed laparoscopic approaches are included with as many illustrations as possible. Also included are sections on open surgery and the early results from a newer procedure that perhaps might offer a pragmatic compromise approach.

Clearly this text will not be the last work on minimal access hernia repair. However as more and more patients present with a list of detailed questions concerning their prospective operation with information frequently gleaned from the lay media, surgeons will have to consider the operations more openly. The range of options increases almost daily and it is hoped that this text will go some way to assisting the decision making process.

Ara Darzi
John R.T. Monson

Chapter 1
Inguinal hernia: background and history

A. Hill and A. Darzi

Inguinal hernias are among the oldest surgical challenges, having been recognized by the Egyptians (1500 BC) and the Ancient Greeks (Hippocrates, 400 BC). The word hernia is derived from the Greek word *hernios* meaning a bud or offshoot. The incidence of inguinal hernias is difficult to ascertain [1]. Zimmerman and Anson concluded that the prevalence is approximately 5% of the adult male population [2]. A survey from the US Department of Health, Education and Welfare reported a prevalence of 15 per 1000 population [3]. The same survey concluded that 40 million days of restricted activity annually could be attributed to this problem [3]. Overall, adult hernioplasty accounts for approximately 15% (500 000) of general surgery operations annually in the United States [4, 5].

Celsus (AD 40) described Roman surgical practice where taxis was advised for strangulation, trusses for reducible hernia and operations only for pain. The approach was through a scrotal incision and the wound was allowed to granulate. Scar tissue was considered an optimum replacement for a weak abdominal wall. Advances in hernia surgery during the Middle Ages included a description by Guy de Chauliac, in 1363, in which he distinguished femoral from inguinal hernia [6]. In 1556, Franco suggested using a grooved dissector to facilitate dividing the neck of a strangulated hernia and recommended reducing the contents and closing the defect with linen suture material [7]. The Renaissance was a period during which understanding of the anatomy of inguinal hernia was facilitated by careful cadaveric dissection. In 1721, Cheselden reported operating upon a patient with a strangulated inguinal hernia who survived to return to work [8]. However, there were less fortunate individuals during the history of hernia surgery. Cheselden also describes some patients who survived a strangulated hernia only to develop a faecal fistula [8]. Sir Percival Pott, who was probably the first to suggest the congenital origin of hernias, described the pathophysiology of a strangulated inguinal hernia in 1757 [9].

Early in the nineteenth century, four men contributed important descriptions of inguinal anatomy: Camper [10], Cooper [11], Hesselbach [12, 13] and Scarpa [14]. In 1801, Camper published the description of the fascia that bears his name. The skilled anatomist Sir Astley Cooper (1768–1841) published his two-volume work, *The Anatomy and Surgical Treatment of Abdominal Hernia*, in 1804 and 1807. First descriptions credited to Cooper include transversalis fascia, internal ring, inguinal canal, correct formation of femoral sheath by the transversalis fascia, and the complete description of Camper's fascia. He paid little attention to 'the ligament of pubis', now called Cooper's ligament, and he certainly had no idea how important this structure would become in the modern treatment of hernias. Hesselbach described the triangle that bears his name in 1814, while he was prosector in the Anatomic Theatre of Wurzburg. Finally, in this quartet of anatomists must be included Scarpa, for whom a superficial layer of fascia is named.

The nineteenth century brought anaesthesia, haemostasis and antisepsis, which made modern hernia surgery possible. As in every area of surgery, these advances allowed rapid development of the science of hernia surgery. The discovery by Lister of the nature of sepsis and his introduction of antisepsis in about 1870 was an important landmark during this period [15]. Further landmarks in the development of surgery were the introduction of surgical gloves by Halsted in 1896 and of aseptic technique by von Mickulicz in 1904. Many attempts were made at hernioplasty throughout the years including efforts by Wood (1863) who described subcutaneous division and suture of the sac and fascial separation of the groin from the scrotum [16] and Czerney (1876) who pulled the sac through the external ring and amputated it allowing the neck to spring back to the deep ring [17]. Kocher (1907), who was the first surgeon to win the Nobel prize, described invagination and fixation of the sac laterally to the external oblique muscle [18]. Not surprisingly, none of these procedures survived the test of time. One wonders with the advent of laparoscopic surgery whether laparoscopic repair is yet another technique to add to this lengthy list of failed hernioplasties.

Two surgeons made outstanding contributions to the development of hernia surgery during the nineteenth century—the American Marcy (1871) [19] and the Italian Bassini (1884) [20, 21]. Both surgeons were noted for their understanding of the anatomy of the inguinal canal, how each anatomic plane, transversalis fascia, transverse and oblique muscles, and the external oblique aponeurosis contributed to the canal's stability. Edoardo Bassini of the Padua clinic in Italy is given the deserved accolade as the father of modern hernia surgery. Born in 1844, in Pavia, Italy, he was the first to perform a true herniorrhaphy (in 1884). The Bassini repair involves bringing transversus abdominus aponeurosis rather than muscle fibres down to Poupart's ligament. Bassini emphasized this point, although it has often been unwisely ignored by surgeons doing this type of repair. Bassini's technique has stood the test of time and remains today the standard against which the repair of inguinal hernias is judged. In 1889, in a masterful surgical treatise, Bassini reported an incidence of recurrence well under 10%, with only one death in 262 hernia repairs. This report indeed shook the surgical world, which was accustomed to a mortality rate of 6–7% and recurrences of at least 40–50% within a year—this from fine surgical centres such as Billroth's clinic.

However, credit for modern herniotomy should be given to Marcy, a native of Massachusetts and a pupil of Lister. He first described closure of the internal ring with carbolized catgut sutures. An operation performed by Marcy in 1869 and reported in 1871 pre-dated Bassini by almost 15 years. In 1881, Bassini heard the report, in which Marcy expertly described the anatomy of the internal ring, the high ligation of the sac, and the importance of the obliquity of the canal and the transversalis fascia. The teachings of Marcy were not widely accepted, and it remained for Bassini, using Marcy's technique as a guide, to effect the revolution in the surgical treatment of hernia.

In 1889, William Halsted, unaware of Bassini's report, described a single case in which he had used a procedure independently devised. His procedure was startling in its similarity to the Bassini repair; this he later acknowledged. The Halsted and Bassini procedures differed mainly in that the former placed the spermatic cord superficial to the external oblique fascia, while the latter placed it deep to that same structure. This latter description was known as the Halsted I repair. A further modification to this procedure was described in 1893 and became known as the Halsted II repair in which the creation of an aponeurotic flap from the anterior rectus sheath is used to reinforce the repair. He did not, however, discover the value of a relaxing incision in the anterior rectus sheath, which was first described by Wolfler in 1892. Halsted popularized its use in 1903 but the European literature mistakenly credits Tanner with its introduction.

A.H. Ferguson (1899) was responsible for the next notable development in hernia repair when he advised against any mobilization of the cord: 'Tearing the cord out of its bed is without an anatomic reason to recommend it, a physiologic act to suggest it, an aetiologic factor in hernia to suggest it, nor brilliant surgical results to justify its continuance. Leave the cord alone, for it is the sacred highway along which travel vital elements indispensible to the perpetuity of our race'. Ferguson sutured the fascia transversalis lateral to the deep ring, then, leaving the cord undisturbed, he drew the internal oblique down in front of the cord and sutured it to the inguinal ligament [22].

After the nineteenth century advances of Marcy and Bassini, and the important contribution to surgical technique by Halsted, little of major importance was contributed until the 1920s. Countless other modifications of Marcy's and Bassini's operations were made and reported frequently, with no adequate outcome measures. Alternatives to the anterior (inguinal) approach to the internal ring include the transabdominal (laparotomy) and the extraperitoneal (preperitoneal) approach. Lawson Tait recommended midline abdominal section for umbilical and groin hernia in 1891 [23]. LaRoque, in 1919, recommended transabdominal repair of inguinal hernias through a muscle-splitting incision about one inch above the internal ring [24].

The extraperitoneal–preperitoneal approach owes its origin to Cheatle (1920) who initially used a midline incision (1920) but subsequently (1921) changed to a Pfannenstiel incision [25, 26]. Cheatle explored both sides, and inguinal and femoral protrusions were reduced and amputated. If needed, for strangulation or adhesions, the peritoneum could easily be opened. The fascia transversalis was visible and easily repaired. Cheatle advised against this approach for direct hernia because the direct region was usually obscured and distorted by the retraction of the rectus muscles. A.K. Henry rediscovered and popularized the extraperitoneal approach in 1936 [27].

In 1923 Gallie and Le Mesurier described their method of repair with strips of fascia lata. In this repair strips of fascia from the thigh were used to strengthen the posterior wall of the inguinal canal. Gallie claimed good results with his 'fascial darn' and the article that he co-wrote with his colleague Le Mesurier [28] did much to popularize his operation in the clinics at home and abroad. In other hands, however, Gallie's operation left much to be desired. The recurrence rate was high: 8–10%. Again the needle employed for the lattice repair was large and cumbersome and traumatized the inguinal ligament and also the muscular layers through which it had to be passed. The long scar in the thigh or the gap in the ileotibial band produced by the fasciotomy in some cases gave trouble. This was particularly brought to light in World War II, when a number of servicemen had to be invalided from active service on account of alleged pain in the scar in the thigh.

Modern hernia repair is associated with excellent results from specialist centres such as the Shouldice Clinic. No history of hernia surgery would be complete without mention of the contribution of Earle Shouldice and his colleagues in Toronto, who have collected and evaluated data on many thousands of patients [29–31]. The Shouldice Clinic has a remarkably low recurrence rate of 0.6% for over 6000 hernia repairs with a minimum follow-up of 10 years [32]. One feature of this type of hernia repair is that it is easily exported from the specialist clinic to the practice of many surgeons throughout the world. The combined experience of several surgeons using the Shouldice repair on over 22 000 hernias has resulted in a recurrence rate of 1.3% [33]. However, hernia surgery is still associated with recurrence rates of between 16 and 35% when all types of hernia repair are evaluated. Devlin has suggested that inadequate follow-up of many published series may explain a higher true recurrence rate than that commonly reported in the literature [34].

Traditional inguinal hernia repair is not without complications such as division of the ilioinguinal, iliohypogastric and both the genital and femoral branches of the genitofemoral nerve. The testicular blood supply may be impaired resulting in testicular atrophy. Swelling of the testis due to trauma to the venous or lymphatic vessels of the cord or 'too tight' a repair are other recognized complications. In an attempt to avoid some of these complications, primary inguinal hernia repair using prosthetic mesh was introduced and was popularized by Rives [35] and Stoppa *et al.* [36]. Lichtenstein *et al.* [37] suggested a tension-free repair of the posterior wall of the inguinal canal by inserting a prosthetic mesh extraperitoneally to create a new inguinal floor. They suggested that pain, the complications resulting from an overtight repair, and recurrence rates would all be reduced. A recent report by Lichtenstein involving over 3000 patients has shown a recurrence rate of only 0.5% [38].

It appears that the technique of hernia repair is still under development despite several centuries of progress. Convalescence time away from work after hernia surgery remains an important loss of income to both individual and nation [39]. It is now generally accepted that the patient should return to work within 4 weeks of an uncomplicated inguinal hernia repair [39–42]. Laparoscopic hernia repair heralds a new era in hernia surgery with the potential to reduce this recovery period further. Laparoscopic surgeons have applied Lichtenstein's principle of a tension-free hernioplasty using a transperitoneal approach. The preperitoneal placement of a mesh is also performed laparoscopically. Whether laparoscopic repair of inguinal hernias stands the test of time remains to be seen. The last chapter in the history of groin anatomy and operative repair of hernia defects has yet to be written.

References

1 Nyhus LM, Condon RE. *Hernia*, 2nd edn. JB Lippincott, Philadelphia, 1978.
2 Zimmerman IM, Anson BJ. *The Anatomy and Surgery of Hernia*, 2nd edn. Williams and Wilkins, Baltimore, 1967.

3 US Department of Health, Education and Welfare. *National Health Survey on Hernias*, series B, No. 25, December 1960.
4 Lichtenstein IL. *Hernia Repair Without Disability*, 2nd edn. Ishiyaku Euroamerica Inc, St Louis, 1986.
5 Berliner SD. An approach to groin hernia. *Surg Clin North Am* 1984; **64**: 197–213.
6 de Chauliac G. *La Grande Chirurgie composée en 1363. Revue avec des notes, une introduction sur le moyenage. Sur la vie et les oeuvres de Guy de Chauliac par E. Nicaise.* Felix Alcan, Paris, 1890.
7 Franco P. *Traites des hernies contenant une ample declaration de toutes leurs especes et autre excellentes parties de la chirurgie, assauoir de la pierre, des cataractes des yeux, et autre maladies, desquelles comme la cure est perilleuse, aussi est elle de peu d'hommes bien exercee.* Thibauld Payan, Lyon, 1561.
8 Cheselden W. *The Anatomy of the Human Body*, 12th edn. Livingstone, Dodsley, Cadell, Baldwin and Lowndes, London, 1784.
9 Pott P. *Treatise on Ruptures.* Hitch and Hawes, London, 1757.
10 Camper P. *Icones Herniarum.* Francforti ad Moenum, Varrentrapp and Wenner, 1801.
11 Cooper AP. *The Anatomy and Treatment of Abdominal Hernia.* 2 volumes. Longman and Co., London, 1804–7.
12 Hesselbach FK. *Anatomisch-chirurgische Abhandlung uber den Ursprung der Leistenbruke.* Baumgarten, Wurzburg, 1806.
13 Hesselbach FK. *Nueste anatomisch-pathologische Untersuchungen uber den Ursprung und das Forschreiten der Leisten und Schenkel-bruche.* Baumgarten, Wurzburg, 1814.
14 Scarpa A. *Sull'ernia del revineo.* P. Bizzoni, Pavia, 1821.
15 Lister J. Note on the preparation of catgut for surgical purposes. *Br Med J* 1908; **i**: 125–126.
16 Read RC. The development of inguinal herniorrhaphy. *Surg Clin North Am* 1984; **64**: 185–196.
17 Czerny V. Studien zur Radikalbehandlung der Hernien. *Wiener Medizinische Wochenschrift* 1877; **27**: 497–500.
18 Kocher T. *Chirurgische Operationslehre.* Verlag von Gustav Fischer, Jena, 1907.
19 Marcy HO. The cure of hernia. *JAMA* 1887; **8**: 589–592.
20 Bassini E. Nuova technica per la cura radicale dell'ernia. *Atti del Associazione Medica Italiano Congresso* 1887; **2**: 179–182.
21 Bassini E. Nuova technica per la cura dell'ernia inguinali. *Societa Italiana di Chirurgica* 1887; **4**: 379–382.
22 Ferguson AH. Oblique inguinal hernia. Typic operation for its radical cure. *JAMA* 1899; **33**: 6–14.
23 Tait L. A discussion on treatment of hernia by median abdominal section. *Br Med J* 1891; **ii**: 685–691.
24 LaRoque GP. The permanent cure of inguinal and femoral hernia. A modification of standard operative procedures. *Surg Gynaecol Obstet* 1919; **29**: 507–511.
25 Cheatle GL. An operation for radical cure of inguinal and femoral hernia. *Br Med J* 1920; **ii**: 68–69.
26 Cheatle GL. An operation for inguinal hernia. *Br Med J* 1921; **ii**: 1025–1026.
27 Henry AK. Operation for femoral hernia by a midline extraperitoneal approach: with a preliminary note on the use of this route for reducible inguinal hernia. *Lancet* 1936; **i**: 531–533.
28 Gallie WE, Le Mesurier AB. Living sutures in the treatment of hernia. *Can Med Assoc J* 1923; **13**: 468–480.
29 Shouldice EE. Obesity and ventral repair. *Modern Medicine of Canada* 1953, Aug 89.
30 Shouldice EE. The treatment of hernia. *Ontario Med Rev* 1953: 1–14.
31 Shouldice EE, Glassow F, Black N. Sinus formation following infected herniorrhaphy incisions. *Can Med Assoc J* 1961; **84**: 576–579.
32 Glassow F. Short stay surgery (Shouldice technique) for repair of inguinal hernia. *Ann R Coll Surg Engl* 1976; **58**: 133–139.
33 Glassow F. Inguinal hernia repair using local anaesthesia. *Ann R Coll Surg Engl* 1984; **66**: 382–387.
34 Devlin HB. *Management of Abdominal Hernias.* Butterworths, London, 1988: 101–105.
35 Rives J. Surgical treatment of the inguinal hernia by the Dacron patch. Principles, indications, technique and results. *Int Surg* 1967; **47**: 360–364.
36 Stoppa RE, Rives JL, Worlaumont C. The use of dacron in the repair of hernias of the groin. *Surg Clin North Am* 1984; **64**: 269–286.
37 Lichtenstein IL, Shulman AG, Amid PK. The tension free hernioplasty. *Am J Surg* 1989; **157**: 188–193.
38 Shulman AG, Amid PK, Lichtenstein IL. The safety of mesh repair for primary inguinal hernia—results of 3019 operations from five diverse surgical sources. *Am Surg* 1992; **58**: 255–257.
39 Glassow F. Surgical repair of inguinal and femoral hernias. *Can Med Assoc J* 1973; **108**: 308–313.
40 Bourke JB, Lear PA, Taylor M. The effect of early return to work after elective repair of inguinal hernia: clinical and financial consequences at one year and three years. *Lancet* 1981; **ii**: 623–625.
41 Taylor EW, Dewar AP. Early return to work after repair of unilateral inguinal hernia. *Br J Surg* 1983; **70**: 599–600.
42 Semmence A, Kynch J. Hernia repair and time off work in Oxford. *J R Coll Gen Pract* 1980; **30**: 90–96.

Chapter 2

Open repair of groin hernias

A.D. Spigelman

In this chapter I deal with traditional or open methods of *elective* groin hernia repair in adults. In respect of inguinal hernias, there are many repairs to choose from, suggesting that we are still to find the ideal method of herniorrhaphy. Perhaps this perceived failure has provided the impetus for the advent of the laparoscopic approach, although 'market forces' (used in the broadest sense) have also had an important role to play. Have we, however, really failed to reach a truly 'gold standard' in the repair of inguinal hernias? Or do unacceptably high recurrence rates reflect a disinclination among surgeons to learn and to adopt one of the two procedures that have reported the lowest recurrence rates [1]?

Indications for surgery

Inguinal hernia

All inguinal hernias should be repaired, with the exception of small and easily reduced direct hernias. If in doubt as to the nature of the hernia (that is, direct or indirect), then herniography should allow the correct diagnosis to be made.

In terms of allocating priority to patients, the study of Gallegos *et al.* [2] suggests that patients with a short history of herniation are at greater risk of strangulation than others and should therefore undergo early surgery. This is at odds with the policy of Her Majesty's Government in the United Kingdom (from the 1980s up to the present at least), where political embarrassment has produced a system in which patients at the end of a waiting list are given priority. This works to the detriment of hernia patients in other ways; when central funding produced a series of 'Waiting List Initiatives' there was a fall in the proportion of low-priority varicose vein patients at the expense of hernia patients, the proportion of whom rose when this process was audited in rural England [3].

Femoral hernia

Although accounting for about one-tenth of groin hernias, femoral hernias are significantly more prone to strangulation [2]. Unobstructed femoral hernias must be repaired within a short time (days, not months) after diagnosis.

Methods

Anaesthesia

Local anaesthesia is preferred in all but very anxious or obese patients, or those with large hernias that might require much dissection and traction. This mode of anaesthesia dictates more delicate handling of tissues, thereby reducing trauma [4]. It is also associated with a lower risk for postoperative urinary retention than is general or spinal anaesthesia [5, 6].

Spinal or general anaesthesia is used in those patients unsuitable for the local anaesthetic technique.

Before injecting the local anaesthetic solution, lignocaine and prilocaine (EMLA) cream is applied along the line of incision. I use a cocktail of 20 ml of 1% lignocaine with adrenaline and 10 ml of plain bupivacaine with 20 ml of normal saline added for volume and 5 ml of 8.4% sodium bicarbonate to increase the pH of the solution. This latter step eliminates the stinging that can otherwise cause discomfort upon injection of the anaesthetic [7], which can also be reduced by warming the solution to 37°C [8]. Bupivacaine also provides postoperative pain relief; however, ropivacaine could be substituted for bupivacaine in order to obviate the latter's potential for cardiotoxicity, while still preserving the use of a long-acting agent [9].

Anaesthetic is injected along the line of incision and deeply, as well as medial to the anterior superior iliac spine in order to block the ilioinguinal nerve. In the case of inguinal hernia repair, further injections are given after making the incision, just deep to the external oblique muscle—so as to flood the cord—and around the neck of the sac.

Use of 0.5% lignocaine with adrenaline alone has also been shown to be safe and effective, particularly in the groin, where absorption of local anaesthetic is relatively slow—perhaps related to the low blood flow of this area [10].

Repeated enquiries are made of the patient; if the patient complains of pain, further anaesthetic is given.

Local anaesthetic may be supplemented by short-acting intravenous sedation (sedoanalgesia).

Inguinal hernia repair

Although about 100 techniques for repair of inguinal hernias have been described [11], and the Bassini and darn techniques are very well known, they are (in developed countries) of historical interest only. This is because the transversalis repair popularized by the Shouldice Clinic in Toronto, Canada [11, 12], and the tension-free mesh hernioplasty promoted by Irving Lichtenstein [13, 14] have the lowest recurrence rates.

The reader will probably already be familiar with the options for open repair of inguinal hernias, and, in hoping to glean information about the advancing front of laparoscopic repair, may wish to skim over this chapter. Indeed, the main value of this book is to document the state of the art at a certain point in time. Actual techniques are learnt best by watching (both live and videoed) operations, and then performing them under tuition on several occasions. This applies to both open and closed methods of hernia repair. Given that proviso, and given that there are ample descriptions of the best methods of open hernia repair already in the literature, there follows a brief account of techniques for the Shouldice and for the tension-free repairs of inguinal hernias. Note that both attend to the back wall—simple inguinal herniotomy in the adult is an inadequate operation.

Beginning the operation (Shouldice and tension-free techniques). All patients should be monitored by pulse oximetry and cardiac chest leads peroperatively. A transverse incision in a skin crease (if available) is preferred.

Having made the incision, branches of the superficial epigastric vessels often require ligation and division (on the lateral aspect of the wound). Camper's and Scarpa's fasciae and then the external oblique muscle are incised. Haemostasis must be meticulous throughout the procedure. The ilioinguinal nerve is identified and placed behind one of the leaves of this muscle (Fig. 2.1). The cremaster muscle and fascia are dissected free and usually divided between clamps, in order to facilitate repair of the back wall. The spermatic cord is elevated either by an encircling instrument or by a tape. If a lipoma of the cord is found then it should be excised (Fig. 2.2). An indirect hernial sac will be apparent anterosuperior to the cord. It is dissected off the cord up to the deep inguinal ring. It is then opened (Fig. 2.3) and transfixed (Fig. 2.4). A co-existing femoral hernia is always checked for and repaired.

Attention is now turned to the back wall. If the patient is awake (local or spinal anaesthesia) then he or she is asked to cough, in order to assess the integrity of the back wall.

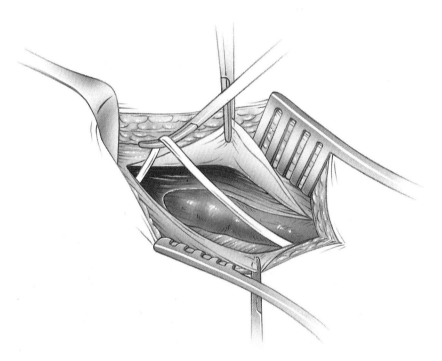

Figure 2.1
Identify the ilioinguinal nerve, which is protected by displacing it behind one of the leaves of the external oblique muscle.

Shouldice technique. The transversalis fascia is incised (Fig. 2.5) after separating it from the extraperitoneal fat on which it lies. The transversalis fascia is then reconstituted using a four-layer overlapping technique (with 2/0 Prolene—a modification of the original Shouldice technique, in which wire was used). The first of the four layers is begun medially at the pubic tubercle, suturing the lower flap of transversalis fascia to the underside of the upper flap, using a continuous stitch (Fig. 2.6). The internal ring is reached and tightened, but not overly so. The running suture is then brought back

Figure 2.2
Excision of cord lipoma.

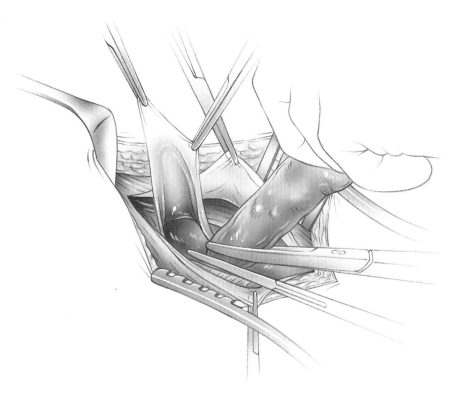

Figure 2.3
An empty open indirect sac.

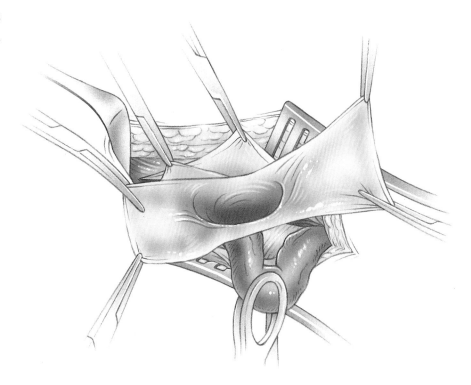

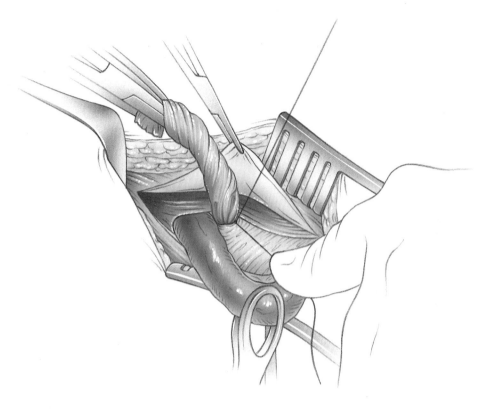

Figure 2.4
Herniotomy—transfixion of the sac.

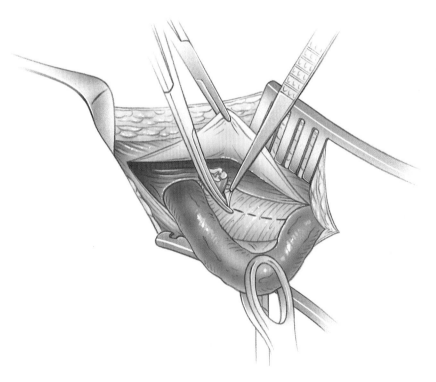

Figure 2.5
Line of incision of transversalis fascia (Shouldice inguinal hernia repair).

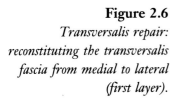

Figure 2.6
*Transversalis repair:
reconstituting the transversalis
fascia from medial to lateral
(first layer).*

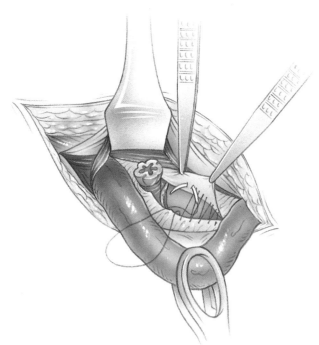

medially, tacking the free end of the superior leaf of the transversalis fascia to the upturned deep edge of the inguinal ligament (where the lower leaf of transversalis fascia condenses with the inguinal ligament), finally being tied to the end of the suture that was left long initially. The next two layers are started laterally, just medial to the internal ring. Another 2/0 Prolene stitch is used, bringing down the underside of the conjoint tendon to the inguinal ligament (Fig. 2.7). Once the pubic tubercle area is reached, the suture is brought back laterally, approximating the conjoint tendon to the external oblique aponeurosis, just above the inguinal ligament, until

Figure 2.7
*Transversalis repair:
reconstituting the transversalis
fascia from lateral to medial
(third layer).*

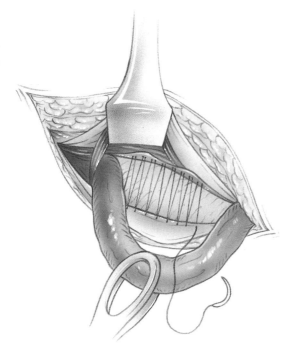

the deep ring is reached. The two ends of the suture are then tied. The repair is tested by asking the patient to cough.

Closure is in layers, with a subcuticular absorbable suture and/or adhesive skin strips being used in the skin, in order to eliminate the need for suture removal [15].

Mesh technique. Whereas the Shouldice technique relies on overlapping reinforcing layers, each one in theory taking tension off the others, the mesh method avoids the use of tension entirely.

A sheet of polypropylene mesh (the same material that goes to make Prolene sutures) is fashioned to size, with a slit creating two tails around the lateral end of the cord. Polypropylene mesh is chosen because it is well tolerated, does not increase the risk of infection and fixes itself well to host tissue, into which it is readily incorporated [16]. It also provides superior tensile strength compared with other types of mesh [17].

The mesh is placed in the floor of the inguinal canal, overlapping the pubic tubercle by 1–2 cm. A continuous 2/0 Prolene suture is applied between the lower border of the mesh and the upturned deep edge of the inguinal ligament, finishing at the beginning of the pre-cut mesh tails. A single suture tacks the upper tail over the lower tail and onto the inguinal ligament, lateral to the deep inguinal ring. The upper edge of the mesh is sutured to the conjoint tendon with loosely applied interrupted Prolene sutures. This completes the repair; further steps are as described for the Shouldice technique. Drains are not usually necessary for either technique.

Femoral hernia repair

Low, high or higher? That is the question. 'Low' (or crural) means an approach inferior to the inguinal ligament, over the hernia itself; 'high' alludes to repair via the inguinal canal (with concomitant damage to that canal); while 'higher' refers to the higher skin incision used in the preperitoneal or extraperitoneal approach. The principles of repair remain constant regardless of approach; that is, find the defect, isolate the sac, deal with its contents, close, transfix and remove the sac, reduce the sac remnant, and repair the defect through which the sac prolapsed. The bladder should be catheterized prior to surgery, in order to reduce the risk posed by the bladder sliding onto the medial sac wall. The sac is therefore opened on its lateral aspect to avoid inadvertent damage to the bladder.

The operation chosen will depend on the surgeon's experience and the patient's build—hernia in a thin patient being relatively easy to repair using the low approach. However, the conventional counsel of excellence dictates use of the preperitoneal ('higher') approach, which, although not usually suitable for local anaesthesia, affords an excellent view of structures involved and allows for easy repair of bilateral femoral hernias. The skin incision is a transverse one and is made about 3 cm above the inguinal ligament. After cutting through the subcutaneous tissue, the anterior rectus sheath is incised transversely; this incision is extended laterally and deeply so as to expose the transversalis fascia. The rectus muscle is then retracted medially, the transversalis fascia is incised and blunt dissection is employed to push away the preperitoneal fat. It should now be possible to see the hernial sac disappearing down through the femoral canal (Fig. 2.8).

Figure 2.8

The view obtained using the preperitoneal approach for femoral hernia repair.

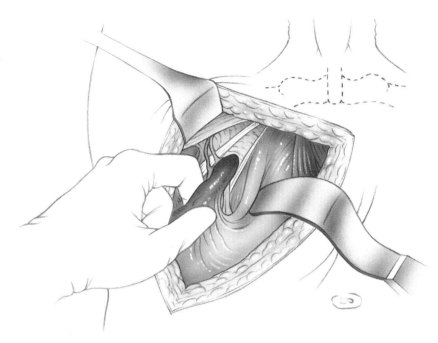

Although the low approach is suitable for nearly all elective femoral hernia repairs, unless the preperitoneal approach is used in elective cases, unfamiliarity with the anatomy encountered when using the preperitoneal approach will mean that it will not be used on those occasions when it is most useful: namely, in the emergency situation where gangrenous bowel might be present. Otherwise, when bowel resection is required, another incision, usually entailing formal laparotomy, will be needed—unless, of course, one is able to convert to a laparoscopic approach.

The inguinal canal approach should probably only be used when there is a coexisting inguinal hernia to repair.

Closure of the defect is by approximation of the inguinal ligament to the pectineal ligament using a Prolene suture or two, usually (low approach) with an overlying supporting patch of the fascia which lies superficial to and has been dissected off the pectineus muscle. Partial occlusion of the femoral vein at the lateral aspect of the repair by the suture should be avoided. A Prolene mesh plug may be fashioned, inserted into the femoral canal and held in place by sutures as another way to close the defect [18].

Day case or not?

Day-case surgery is considerably more popular in the United States than in the United Kingdom. Although it is recommended that *at least* 30% of elective groin herniorrhaphies in the United Kingdom be performed on a day-case basis [19], only 7% are presently carried out as day cases [20].This is despite the fact that nearly four decades have elapsed since it was shown that groin hernias could be safely and effectively repaired on a day-case basis (that is, with the patient being admitted and discharged on the day of operation) [21]. Furthermore, over three decades ago Stephens and Dudley [22] outlined the community care necessary to run such a service, while clinical outcome was shown to be good nearly two decades ago [23, 24].

Nevertheless, considerable variation remains in rates of day-care surgery for hernias between countries [25], within individual countries [26] and even within the same hospital [27]. This last point reflects the large variation in surgeons' attitudes to day-case surgery [28], although duration of hospital stay is not related to the probability of recurrence [29]. While some studies show good patient satisfaction with day-case repair [30], others report problems [31].

Selection of suitable patients for day-care surgery

Patients should be healthy or have only mild systemic disease. Patients with serious systemic disease may be suitable for local anaesthesia, but it is prudent to admit such patients for monitoring. Information given to the patient in the clinic should consist of a written information sheet explaining the diagnosis, preoperative instructions, principles of the operation and postoperative care.

A patient questionnaire, previously agreed to by the anaesthetist, should be completed, so that the patient's fitness for day-care surgery can be determined, as well as clarifying which, if any, preoperative investigations are necessary. Finally, the patient's social circumstances (e.g. housing, help at home) must be satisfactory for the procedure to be done as a day case.

Postoperative care

After a period of observation on the day-care unit, patients are discharged in the company of another adult. Ideally, a district nurse visits on the night of (or morning after) surgery. The patient is told to contact the operating hospital in the first instance rather than the family doctor in the event of any early problems.

Patients should be supplied with adequate analgesia; laxatives are recommended to avoid constipation.

Return to social and physical activity should be within days of surgery. Return to work depends on the nature of the work but should be by 2 weeks for all except those in heavy work, who should be fit to work by 4 weeks. Most patients can in fact return to work earlier than these guidelines indicate.

One postoperative visit to the surgeon is recommended.

Complications and how to minimize them

Wound haematoma formation and bruising can be minimized by scrupulous haemostasis and gentle handling of tissues. Ischaemic orchitis and atrophy of the testis can be avoided in the same way, and also by leaving a distal indirect sac in place. Wound infection rates can be reduced by avoidance of braided sutures, removing hair over the wound immediately preoperatively *only* [32], use of a depilatory cream for this, showering of the patient before operation and use of povidone-iodine as skin preparation.

Damage to the ilioinguinal nerve is minimized by protecting it as outlined above.

All patients should receive prophylaxis for deep venous thrombosis: namely, leg compression stockings, subcutaneous heparin (to commence before surgery) and early mobilization.

Recurrence can be minimized by adequate training in technical aspects, use of non-absorbable suture material as outlined, and complete dissection so as to avoid missing a hernia.

Audit

Regardless of the mode of repair, results should be monitored regularly. Measurements should include postoperative morbidity (such as infection, urinary retention), recurrence and patient satisfaction.

Postoperative complications should be assessed by surveillance in the community as well as by assessment at the postoperative visit. Otherwise most wound problems will go unrecognized [33].

Conclusion

Both of the operations for inguinal hernia, as outlined in this chapter, that give the best results, can be done under local anaesthetic in most cases, and most can be done on a day-care or 'ambulatory' basis [7]. Why, then, pursue other techniques when the 5-year recurrence rates of these two procedures fall well below 0.5%, deemed acceptable by the Royal College of Surgeons of England [19]?

Perhaps the answer lies not in the recurrence rate, but in other factors such as the incidence of wound infection, ilioinguinal nerve damage and the time taken to return to work. Yet wound infections as well as ilioinguinal nerve damage occur with both laparoscopic and open techniques [34]. It might be expected that the omission of a larger incision would promote early return to normal activities, as, for instance, in laparoscopic cholecystectomy versus the open method. However, early ambulation and return to work are also encouraged by the Shouldice herniorrhaphy and by the tension-free mesh hernioplasty. Another factor favouring the laparoscopic approach might be its ability to deal with bilateral hernias without producing additional wounds. However, although some counsel against open repair of bilateral inguinal hernia simultaneously, on the grounds of increased morbidity and an increased recurrence rate [19, 35], others dispute this [36]. Thus, even here, there is no clear winner.

What about repair of recurrent inguinal hernias? In the case of a patient with a recurrent inguinal hernia initially repaired using an open approach, it is relatively simple to open the old wound and repair such a recurrence by using a plug of mesh [37]. Although laparoscopic hernia repair has the advantage of allowing the operator to avoid transgressing the old operative field, reducing the risk of damaging the spermatic cord structures, so too does the open preperitoneal approach reported by Nyhus *et al.* [38].

The true explanation for the advance of laparoscopic herniorrhaphy is probably irrelevant anyway, and may relate to fashion and to 'manufacturers extravagant support' [39] as much as anything else. Whether the laparoscopic approach is superior in terms of any of the criteria mentioned above clearly awaits the outcome of randomized studies.

Finally, be wary of the reason for development of an inguinal hernia. It may be related to straining when voiding (therefore, fix the prostate problem first); or it may be related to straining at stool, so have a low threshold for examining the bowel. Indeed, Lovett *et al.* [40] found colorectal pathology in the majority of 464 asymptomatic male patients over 40 years of age presenting with inguinal hernias by performing flexible sigmoidoscopy; cancer was found in 22 patients and premalignant (adenomatous) polyps in 97 patients.

References

1 Morgan M, Swan AV, Reynolds A, Beech R, Devlin HB. Are current techniques of inguinal hernia repair optimal? A survey in the United Kingdom. *Ann R Coll Surg Engl* 1991; **73**: 341–345.
2 Gallegos NC, Dawson J, Jarvis M, Hobsley M. Risk of strangulation in groin hernias. *Br J Surg* 1991; **78**: 1171–1173.
3 Umeh HN, Reece-Smith H, Faber RG, Galland RB. Impact of a waiting list initiative on a general surgical waiting list. *Ann R Coll Surg Engl* 1994; **76** (Suppl): 4–7.
4 Deysine M, Grimson RC, Soroff HS. Inguinal herniorrhaphy: reduced morbidity by service standardisation. *Arch Surg* 1991; **126**: 628–630.
5 Finley RK, Miller SF, Jones LM. Elimination of urinary retention following inguinal herniorrhaphy. *Am Surg* 1991; **57**: 486–489.
6 Petros JG, Rimm EB, Robillard RJ, Argy O. Factors influencing postoperative urinary retention in patients undergoing elective inguinal herniorrhaphy. *Am J Surg* 1991; **161**: 431–434.
7 Wantz GE. Ambulatory hernia surgery. *Br J Surg* 1989; **76**: 1228–1229.
8 Davidson JAH, Boom SJ. Warming lignocaine to reduce pain associated with injection. *Br Med J* 1992; **305**: 617–618.
9 Marsh CR, Hardy AJ. Ropivacaine: a new local anaesthetic agent. *Br J Hosp Med* 1991; **45**: 94–95.
10 Karatassas A, Morris RG, Walsh D, Hung P, Slavotinek AH. Evaluation of the safety of inguinal hernia repair in the elderly using lignocaine infiltration anaesthesia. *Aust N Z J Surg* 1993; **63**: 266–269.
11 Bendavid R. New techniques in hernia repair. *World J Surg* 1989; **13**: 522–531.
12 Glassow F. Inguinal hernia repair using local anaesthesia. *Ann R Coll Surg Engl* 1984; **66**: 382–387.
13 Lichtenstein IL, Shulman AG, Amid PK, Montllor MM. The tension-free hernioplasty. *Am J Surg* 1989; **157**: 188–193.
14 Shulman AG, Amid PK, Lichtenstein IL. The safety of mesh repair for primary inguinal hernias: results of 3019 operations from five diverse surgical sources. *Am Surg* 1992; **58**: 255–257.
15 Spigelman AD. Inguinal hernia repair. *Update* 1993; **47**: 436–445.
16 Amid PK, Shulman AG, Lichtenstein IL. Selecting synthetic mesh for the repair of groin hernia. *Postgrad Gen Surg* 1992; **4**: 150–155.
17 Tyrell J, Silberman H, Chandrasoma P, Niland J. Absorbable versus permanent mesh in abdominal operations. *Surgery* 1989; **168**: 227–232.
18 Allan SM, Heddle RM. Prolene plug repair for femoral hernia. *Ann R Coll Surg Engl* 1989; **71**: 220–221.
19 Royal College of Surgeons of England—Report of a Working Party: *Clinical Guidelines in the Management of Groin Hernia in Adults.* July 1993.
20 Kingsnorth AN. Tightening up on groin hernia repair. *Hospital Update* 1993; **19**: 579–581.
21 Farquharson EL. Early ambulation with special reference to herniorrhaphy as an outpatient procedure. *Lancet* 1955; **ii**: 517–519.
22 Stephens FO, Dudley HAF. An organisation for out-patient surgery. *Lancet* 1961; **i**: 1042–1044.
23 Russell IT, Fell M, Devlin B *et al.* Day case surgery for hernias and haemorrhoids: a clinical, social and economic evaluation. *Lancet* 1977; **i**: 844–845.
24 Ruckley CV, Cuthbertson C, Fenwick N *et al.* Day care after operations for hernia or varicose veins: a controlled trial. *Br J Surg* 1978; **65**: 456–459.

25 Morgan M, Beech R. Variations in length of stay and rates of day case surgery: implications for the efficiency of surgical management. *J Epidemiol Community Health* 1990; **44**: 90–105.
26 Henderson J, Goldacre MJ, Griffith M, Simmons HM. Day case surgery: geographical variation, trends and readmission rates. *J Epidemiol Community Health* 1989; **43**: 301–305.
27 Spigelman AD. An initial experience of day surgery repair of inguinal hernias. *J One-Day Surg* 1991; **1**: 22–23.
28 Linos DA, Beard CM, O'Fallon WM, Docherty MB, Beart RW, Kurland LT. Cholecystectomy and carcinoma of the colon. *Lancet* 1981; **ii**: 379–381.
29 Devlin HB, Gillen PHA, Waxman BP, MacNay RA. Short stay surgery for inguinal hernia: experience of the Shouldice operation, 1970–1982. *Br J Surg* 1986; **73**: 123–124.
30 Davies AH, Horrocks M. Patient evaluation and complications of day-case herniorrhaphy under local anaesthetic. *J R Coll Surg Edinb* 1989; **34**: 137–139.
31 Michaels JA, Reece-Smith H, Faber RG. Case–control study of patient satisfaction with day-case and inpatient inguinal hernia repair. *J R Coll Surg Edinb* 1992; **37**: 99–100.
32 McIntyre FJ, McCloy R. Leading article—Shaving patients before operation: a dangerous myth? *Ann R Coll Surg Engl* 1994; **76**: 3–4.
33 Bailey IS, Karran SE, Toyn K, Brough P, Ranaboldo C, Karran SJ. Community surveillance of complications after hernia surgery. *Br Med J* 1992; **304**: 469–471.
34 Woods S, Polglase A. Ilioinguinal nerve entrapment from laparoscopic hernia repair. *Aust N Z J Surg* 1993; **63**: 823–824.
35 Miller AR, van Heerden JA, Naessens JM, O'Brien PC. Simultaneous bilateral hernia repair: a case against conventional wisdom. *Ann Surg* 1991; **213**: 272–276.
36 Serpell JW, Jarrett PEM, Johnson CD. A prospective study of bilateral inguinal hernia repair. *Ann R Coll Surg Engl* 1990; **72**: 299–303.
37 Shulman AG, Amid PK, Lichtenstein IL. The 'plug' repair of 1402 recurrent inguinal hernias. *Arch Surg* 1990; **125**: 265–267.
38 Nyhus LM, Pollack R, Bombeck CT, Donahue PE. The preperitoneal approach and prosthetic buttress repair for recurrent hernia. The evolution of a technique. *Ann Surg* 1988; **208**: 733–737.
39 Editorial. Surgical innovation under scrutiny. *Lancet* 1993; **342**: 187–188.
40 Lovett J, Kirgan D, McGregor B. Inguinal herniation justifies sigmoidoscopy. *Am J Surg* 1989; **158**: 615–617.

Chapter 3

Open mesh repair: technique and review of the literature

A. Hill and A. Darzi

Transabdominal preperitoneal laparoscopic hernia repair is based upon the same principles as Lichtenstein's open mesh hernia repair. Lichtenstein performs a tension-free hernia repair via the inguinal approach using a polypropylene mesh inserted anterior to the posterior wall of the inguinal canal.

The extraperitoneal approach to laparoscopic hernia repair is similar in principle to the herniorrhaphy practised by Rene Stoppa and Jean Rives from France. Rives and Stoppa do not use one approach exclusively. They use either a preperitoneal subumbilical medial approach or an inguinal approach and use Dacron as their synthetic mesh. Stoppa usually uses the preperitoneal subumbilical approach and places a wide prosthesis surrounding the hernial sac without fixation of the synthetic material.

Mesh hernioplasty performed during open hernia surgery is similar in principle to the technique of laparoscopic hernia repair in that a synthetic mesh is placed in the groin without tension. This chapter reviews the work of Lichtenstein, Rives and Stoppa in order to evaluate the principles upon which laparoscopic mesh hernia repair is based.

Lichtenstein tension-free repair

Lichtenstein has described and practised a tension-free hernia repair using a polypropylene mesh inserted anterior to the posterior wall of the inguinal canal. In laparoscopic hernia repair, a mesh is inserted behind the posterior wall of the inguinal canal via the laparoscope.

Anatomy

There is an enormous medical literature on hernia repair. Part of the reason for this is that there remains much disagreement regarding the anatomic structure of the groin despite the enormous expenditure of time and effort of many acknowledged anatomists. No attempt is made here to include an exhaustive review of the anatomic literature. However, structures pertinent to the Lichtenstein repair will be discussed.

The transversalis fascia is said to be an important anatomical structure in inguinal hernia repair. However, Halverson and McVay [1] have admitted that 'transversalis fascia is loose areolar tissue with very little tensile strength'. Condon has agreed that transversalis fascia 'possesses little intrinsic strength and by itself is a worthless material as far as the construction of a sound hernial repair is concerned' [2]. Consequently, Lichtenstein argues that one should not attempt to reconstruct the normal anatomic structure when the mere presence of a hernia attests to the deficiency of the canal floor. The groin is the only area of the abdominal wall that is not supported by a musculotendinous barrier. The transversalis fascia is merely connective tissue of little intrinsic strength and should be differentiated from collagen-rich aponeurosis. It is the latter that provides the true support to the abdominal wall.

The use of the conjoint tendon for reconstruction of the posterior wall of the inguinal canal during inguinal herniorrhaphy has been recommended for many years. However, in over 95% of cases, the internal oblique muscle is muscular until it reaches the anterior rectus sheath [2]. There is only one tendinous structure above the canal—the transversus abdominus muscle—whose fibres are aponeurotic from the internal ring to the pubis. It is upon the strength of this structure that the integrity of all hernia repairs must therefore depend.

Pathophysiology

In the groin, the transversalis fascia bridges the space created superiorly by the arching internal oblique and transversus fibres and inferiorly by Poupart's ligament. This key area is the 'Achilles heel' of the groin. It is the only portion of the abdominal wall not protected by a musculoaponeurotic layer; transversalis fascia alone covers it. It is the deterioration of this transversalis fascia or a genetic weakness which predisposes to the development of inguinal hernia. Reconstruction has always depended upon approximating strong aponeurotic tissue above and below the canal floor. Since Bassini performed the first true herniorrhaphy 100 years ago, all repairs regardless of modifications have had one common disadvantage—tension on the suture line. It is this tension which is the cause of suture or tissue disruption and the prime aetiological factor in hernia recurrence.

Technique

Local anaesthesia is utilized by the infiltration technique rather than field block. The latter is time consuming and requires a larger volume of anaesthetic agent. Injection of 8–10 ml of the local anaesthetic agent beneath the external oblique aponeurosis, prior to opening it, serves to flood the inguinal canal and anaesthetizes the three nerves in this anatomical region. A few more injections at the pubic tubercle and at the base of the hernia sac may be required to complete the anaesthesia.

The external oblique muscle is opened in the direction of its fibres, and the lower leaf is freed from the spermatic cord. The spermatic cord with its cremaster covering is freed from the floor of the inguinal canal and the pubic bone for a distance of approximately 2 cm beyond the pubic tubercle. The spermatic cord is grasped with the thumb and forefinger and a 'window' is created just beneath the vas deferens to allow an avascular plane to be developed in the mesentery between the inferior cremaster fibres and the spermatic cord. When elevating the spermatic cord, great care should be taken to include the external spermatic vessels and the genital nerve with the cord. This ensures that the genital nerve is preserved. Cutting or ligating the genital nerve can cause severe postoperative neuralgia around the lateral scrotum and anteromedial portion of the thigh. The ilioinguinal and iliohypogastric nerves are also preserved. The cremasteric fibres are transversely incised at the level of the internal ring, avoiding the nerves. Complete stripping and excision of the cremasteric fibres from the spermatic cord is unnecessary. This may result in injury to the nerves and small blood vessels and kinking of the vas deferens and increase the risk of postoperative neuralgia. It is usually unnecessary to retract the ilioinguinal nerve separately.

Indirect hernial sacs are free from the cord to a point beyond the neck of the sac. Opening the sac allows for digital examination of the femoral ring, and the sac is reinverted into the abdomen without ligation, which may cause more postoperative pain [3]. However, Lichtenstein does state in his description on hernia repair that the indirect sac can be dealt with according to the surgeon's own personal preference [4]. Direct sacs may be inverted by means of a single absorbable purse-string suture (Figs 3.1 and 3.2).

The external oblique aponeurosis is separated from the underlying internal oblique muscle high enough to accommodate a 6–8 cm wide patch that can overlap the internal oblique muscle and aponeurosis by at least 2–3 cm above the upper border of Hesselbach's triangle.

A sheet of prosthetic mesh measuring about 8 × 16 cm is fashioned. If necessary this may be trimmed narrower by 1–2 cm to match the varying sizes of the inguinal floor. The medial end of the mesh is rounded to the shape of the medial border of the inguinal canal. With the cord retracted upwards, utilizing a running suture of non-absorbable monofilament material, the rounded corner is sutured to the aponeurotic tissue over the pubic bone overlapping the bone by 1–2 cm. This is an important step in the repair as failure to overlap this bone may result in recurrences. The lower edge is attached by a continuous suture of 3/0 Prolene which secures the

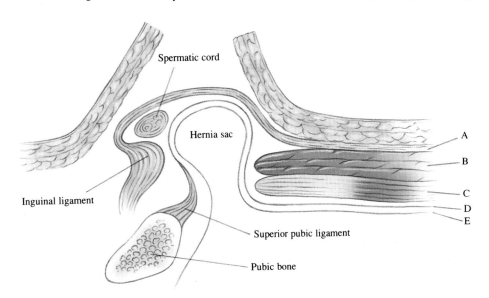

Figure 3.1

A, External oblique aponeurosis. B, Internal oblique muscle. C, Transversus muscle and aponeurosis. D, Transversalis fascia. E, Peritoneum. (From Lichtenstein [4] with permission.)

Figure 3.2

A, External oblique aponeurosis. B, Internal oblique muscle. C, Transversus muscle and aponeurosis. D, Transversalis fascia. E, Peritoneum. (From Lichtenstein [4] with permission.)

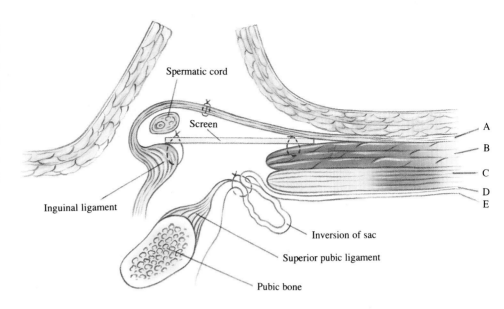

mesh medially to the lacunar ligament and then proceeds laterally along the inguinal ligament beyond the internal ring. A slit in the mesh at the internal ring allows emergence of the spermatic cord. Suturing of the two edges created by this slit to the shelving margin of Poupart's ligament creates a new internal ring made of mesh.

The upper leaf of the external oblique aponeurosis is retracted upward, and the upper edge of the patch is sutured to the internal oblique aponeurosis or muscle, whichever is available (Fig. 3.3) while avoiding injury to or entrapment of the iliohypogastric nerve. Retraction on the upper part of the external oblique aponeurosis is important at this point in the operation in order to achieve the appropriate amount of laxity for the patch. When the retraction is released, the mesh

Figure 3.3

A, Internal oblique muscle. B, Polypropylene screen (mesh). C, External oblique aponeurosis. D, Rectus sheath. E, Inferior cremaster bundle (muscle fibres, genital nerve and vessels) exiting medial to the internal ring. F, Spermatic cord. (From Lichtenstein [4] with permission.)

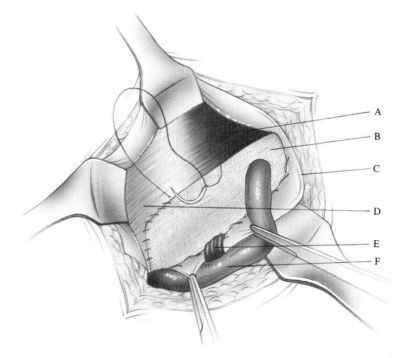

buckles slightly. This desirable laxity ensures a true tension-free repair and is taken up when the patient strains postoperatively.

This alone completes the repair without formal reconstruction of the canal floor. After dusting the wound with antibiotic powder, the external oblique aponeurosis is closed over the cord. Patients are discharged within a few hours of their operation with minimal postoperative pain for which mild analgesics are prescribed. Unrestricted activity is encouraged. Patients resume their normal activities between 2 and 10 days after surgery.

The tension-free repair as described by Lichtenstein is simple and rapid and is associated with less postoperative discomfort and eliminates the prime cause of recurrence. The use of monofilament materials and the addition of local antibiotics virtually eliminate the threat of infection and sinus formation.

Results

Lichtenstein first reported the results of his personal experience of the technique of tension-free hernioplasty for primary inguinal hernias in 1989 [5]. In that paper he reported a series of 1000 patients ranging in age from 1 to 54 years. There were no recurrences; however, he accepted a short follow-up period as being a worthy criticism. A powder of polymyxin and bacitracin had been sprinkled in all wounds. There were two haematomas which resolved spontaneously. No infection was encountered. Over 99% of hernia repairs were performed under local anaesthesia and the patients were able to return home on the day of surgery. All bilateral repairs were handled in the same way and in one sitting. One unusual feature of the population group was the relatively low number of retired elderly men in whom hernias commonly occur. Patients were reported to resume full activity within 2–3 days postoperatively; however, there was no accurate documentation of the number of patients followed, type of work resumed or even the mean follow-up time. The report simply documented a technique. Despite stating that the technique was less painful, no scientific evaluation was performed in terms of visual analogue scales or amount of postoperative analgesia required.

During the next 2 years there were four further publications [6–9] (see Table 3.1) which essentially reported increased numbers of the described technique. Two thousand hernia repairs had been reported by Lichtenstein's group by the end

Year	Journal	No. of cases	Comments
1989 [5]	*Am J Surg*	1000	First report
1990 [6]	*Postgrad Med*	1200	
1990 [8]	*Int Surg*	1500	
1990 [7]	*AORN J*	1500	
1991 [9]	*Am Surg*	2000	
1992 [10]	*Am Surg*	3019	Five surgical centres
1993 [15]	*Am J Surg*	3125	Review of recurrences

Table 3.1
Publications by Lichtenstein on primary inguinal hernia repair using a 'tension-free hernioplasty'.

of 1991, but still all these reports lacked detailed scientific evaluation of the outcome in particular justifying why this procedure was better than other more standard repairs.

In 1992 Lichtenstein's group reported the results from five different surgical centres using the technique of mesh repair for primary inguinal hernias [10]. The other surgeons using the tension-free mesh repair for inguinal hernias included Martin [11], Barnes [12], Capozzi [13] and Tinckler [14]. The results of these 3019 operations are listed in Table 3.2. Their overall failure fate was 0.2%, the infection rate was 0.03%, and there were no reported incidents of mesh rejection. Barnes [12] approximates the transversalis fascia before buttressing his primary repair with a mesh prosthesis, while Capozzi *et al.* [13] 'loosely imbricate the attenuated transversalis fascia' before applying the mesh. Martin [11], Lichtenstein [5] and Tinckler [14] apply the mesh and use it as the sole repair of the floor with no attempt to approximate tissue; thus, they create a true tension-free closure. The follow-up on these studies is now 6 years old [10]. Lichtenstein's two failures were attributed to too small or too tight a patch and failure to place initial sutures beyond the border of the pubic crest. Larger and looser patches have led to a near 100% success rate. This report from five different surgical centres addresses the important issues of recurrence rate, mesh rejection and infection rate [10]. These results appear to imply this is a superior type of hernia repair because of the low infection rate and low recurrence rate with a 5-year follow-up. However, it is necessary to appreciate that this may be the work of five surgeons with an enthusiastic interest in this procedure. There was no explanation given as to how these five centres were chosen to be entered into the study and it might have been said that all centres with bad results were not reported.

Table 3.2

Results of mesh repair of inguinal hernias without formal closure of defect.

Author	Dates	No. of operations	No. of infections	No. of rejections	No. of recurrences
Martin [11]	1976–84	550	0	0	0
Barnes [12]	1976–89	271	0	0	0
Capozzi [13]	1978–88	745	0	0	4
Tinckler [14]	1980–85	392	1	0	3

In 1993 Lichtenstein published a personal series now extending to 3125 hernia repairs with only four recurrences [15]. In addition, in the same work he also reports 23 300 tension-free hernioplasties from 70 different surgical centres having similar data to his own group with regard to postoperative recurrence, rejection and infection rates, as well as postoperative pain and duration of the recovery period [15].

The fact that the results of surgeons without a special interest in hernia repair were identical to those with a special interest in hernia repair is a testimony to the simplicity, safety and effectiveness of open 'tension-free' hernioplasty.

Rives and Stoppa repairs

Jean Rives and Rene Stoppa are French surgeons from Reims and Amiens, respectively, with 30 years of experience in mesh hernia surgery. Both have published extensively in the French literature and to a limited extent in the English literature. Rives and Stoppa do not rule out the use of classic techniques such as the Bassini and McVay procedures. However, they do use prosthetic mesh material in a significant number of their patients. The mesh is inserted deep between the transversalis fascia and the peritoneum in the inguinal or preperitoneal abdominal approach. Rives primarily uses the inguinal approach and Stoppa primarily uses the preperitoneal subumbilical approach.

The Rives inguinal patch

Technique. Primarily using the inguinal approach, Rives inserts a small prosthesis fixed to the parietal wall [16–22]. The surgeon stands on the side of the hernia and proceeds initially as in the Bassini technique. The sac is ligated high and resected. After dividing the transversalis fascia horizontally, the preperitoneal space is dissected with the finger, at first at the top behind the wall, then down behind the horizontal ramus of the pubis. A piece of Dacron mesh, 10 × 10 cm, is fashioned for passage of the spermatic cord. The prosthesis is then stitched down on Cooper's ligament at a distance of 3–4 cm from its inferior edge. The prosthesis is then folded, slipped behind the transversalis fascia, and fixed by several transmuscular stitches. The stitches are placed medially through the rectus abdominus muscle and laterally on both sides of the cord; three or four stitches must be placed on the femoral sheath between the most external point on Cooper's ligament and the most external point on the muscular arch. The prosthesis is thus fixed and tightened moderately without any fold, while the inguinal ring is carried laterally behind the muscles. The transversalis fascia can then be closed in front of the prosthesis, which is hidden under a Bassini-like suture of the fascia and the muscles. The operation is then completed by closing the anterior wall of the canal followed by the skin.

Results. A series of 282 surgical patients with 302 hernias was studied [20, 21]. There were eight infections observed (2.6%) and two recurrences. One hernia recurred after severe sepsis; the other recurrence was caused by an inward disinsertion of the prosthesis. The number of recurrences has not altered for the 143 patients (153 hernias) followed for 2–10 years (1.3%). However, this series is flawed by the low follow-up rate (50.7%).

Stoppa's preperitoneal approach

Technique. Stoppa primarily uses the preperitoneal subumbilical approach [23–27]. The open procedure of preperitoneal mesh repair described by Stoppa is very similar in principle to the extraperitoneal approach to laparoscopic hernia repair. The main aim of preperitoneal mesh repair is the placement of a wide sheet of unresorbable mesh between the muscles and peritoneum. The prosthesis is pressed by intra-abdominal pressure against the inner face of the intra-abdominal wall. By this method, the forces that have themselves created the hernia (that is, pressure of the abdominal contents) are used for repair of the hernia. Stoppa uses Dacron or Mersilene mesh in all his operations.

The surgeon stands on the opposite side to the hernia. A median subumbilical incision is made, and subcutaneous tissue and fascia are divided. The retroparietal dissection commences in the midline in the retropubic space and proceeds laterally and downwards in front of the bladder. The hernial pedicle on the side opposite the operator is isolated. The iliopsoas muscle and the external iliac vessels are safely exposed. Single or multiple hernial sacs are treated in different ways according to their site, volume and degree of adherence to the musculopectineal orifice. Stoppa does not attempt any repair on the hernial orifices. The size of the prosthesis on the patient in question is measured. The correct transverse dimension is equal to the distance between both anterior superior iliac spines minus 2 cm, the height of the prosthesis being equal to the distance between the umbilicus and the pubis. The patch is rectangular, measuring on average 24 cm transversally and 16 cm vertically. The Dacron mesh is placed in the preperitoneal space without excessive tension to surround the visceral sac and overlap the hernial orifices. Occasionally a suction drainage tube is deemed necessary.

Results. Stoppa has reported 255 patients in whom he has performed a preperitoneal mesh hernia repair [28]. A haematoma developed in 8%. The infection rate was 5.8%. 91% of the patients have been followed for 2–10 years post surgery; the recurrence rate was 2.5%. In a more recent update of his work Stoppa reported 572 patients who underwent preperitoneal mesh hernia repair [29]; 3.2% of these patients developed a haematoma and infection occurred in 2.1%. Other complications in this series included chest infection ($n = 7$), phlebitis ($n = 1$) and pulmonary embolus ($n = 1$). The recurrence rate at more than 1 year's follow-up was 1.4%. The reason for these recurrences was that too small Dacron pieces had been used; the recurrence developed by the side of the lower or lateral edge of the mesh. The mean length of hospital stay after preperitoneal repair was 9.7 days. However, this prolonged hospital stay appears to be a feature specific to surgery in France where different economic forces pertain compared with North America.

Discussion

Unlike Lichtenstein, Rives and Stoppa do not recommend the use of Dacron mesh for all hernia repairs. They believe that the risks of infection should limit the use of mesh hernioplasty to men over 50 years, young men who have to return to work promptly, those with bilateral or sliding hernias and obese patients. Although the results of Rives and Stoppa are not as impressive as those of Lichtenstein, they would confirm that in principle the method of mesh hernioplasty should provide an adequate repair of a hernia whether this is performed at open surgery or via the laparoscope. There are many questions that remain to be answered about laparoscopic hernia surgery; however, the principles upon which the repair is based by inserting a polypropylene mesh would appear to be both safe and sound.

References

1 Halverson K, McVay CB. Inguinal and femoral hernioplasty. *Arch Surg* 1970; **101**: 127–135.

2 Nyhus LM, Harkins HM. *Hernia*. JB Lippincott, Philadelphia, 1964: 14–57.

3 Smedberg SGG, Broome AEA, Gullmo A. Ligation of the hernia sac? *Surg Clin North Am* 1984; **64**: 299–306.

4 Lichtenstein IL. *Hernia Repair Without Disability*, 2nd edn. Ishiyaku Euroamerica, Inc., St Louis, 1986: 110–111.

5 Lichtenstein IL, Shulman AG, Amid PK, Montllor MM. The tension free hernioplasty. *Am J Surg* 1989; **157**: 188–193.

6 Lichtenstein IL, Shulman AG, Amid PK. Use of mesh to prevent recurrence of hernias. *Postgrad Med J* 1990; **87**: 155–160.

7 Lichtenstein IL, Shulman AG, Amid PK, Willis PA. Hernia repair with polypropylene mesh. *AORN J* 1990; **52**: 559–565.

8 Lichtenstein IL, Amid PK, Shulman AG. The iliopubic tract. The key to inguinal herniorrhaphy? *Int Surg* 1990; **75**: 244–246.

9 Lichtenstein IL, Shulman AG, Amid PK. Twenty questions about hernioplasty. *Am Surg* 1991; **57**: 730–733.

10 Shulman AG, Amid PK, Lichtenstein IL. The safety of mesh repair for primary inguinal hernias: Results of 3,019 operations from five diverse surgical sources. *Am Surg* 1992; **58**: 255–257.

11 Martin RE, Max CC. Primary inguinal hernia repair with prosthetic mesh. *Hospi Medica* 1984; **1**(3): 1–2.

12 Barnes JP. Inguinal hernia repair with routine use of Marlex mesh. *Surg Gynecol Obstet* 1987; **165**: 33–37.

13 Capozzi JA, Berkenfield JA, Cherry JK. Repair of inguinal hernia in the adult with Prolene mesh. *Surg Gynecol Obstet* 1988; **167**: 124–128.

14 Tinckler LF. Inguinal hernia repair using local anaesthesia. *Ann R Coll Surg Engl* 1985; **67**(4): 268.

15 Amid PK, Shulman AG, Lichtenstein IL. Critical scrutiny of the open 'tension-free' hernioplasty. *Am J Surg* 1993; **165**: 369–371.

16 Rives J. Surgical treatment of the inguinal hernia with Dacron patch. *Int Surg* 1967; **47**: 360–361.

17 Rives J, Nicaise H, Lardennois B. A propos du traitement chirurgical des hernies de l'aine. Orientation nouvelle et perspectives therapeutiques. *Ann Med Pharm (Reims)* 1965; **2**: 193–200.

18 Rives J, Stoppa R, Fortesa L. Les pieces en Dacron et leur place dans la chirurgie des hernies de l'aine. *Ann Chir* 1968; **22**: 159–171.

19 Rives J, Lardennois B, Hibon J. Traitement moderne des hernies de l'aine et de leur recidives. *Paris, Encyclopaedia Medico Chirurgicale, Techniques Chirurgicales*, appareil digestif 1973; **1**(40110): 1–12.

20 Rives J, Lardennois B, Flament JB. La piece en tulle de Dacron, traitement de choix des hernies de l'aine de l'adulte. *Chirurgie* 1973; **99**: 564–575.

21 Rives J, Fortesa L, Drouard F. La voie d'abord abdominale sous-peritoneale dans le traitement des hernies de l'aine. Son histoire, ses indications, ses limites. A propos de 104 observations. *Ann Chir* 1978; **32**: 245.

22 Rives J, Flament JB, Delattre JF. La Chirurgie moderne des hernies de l'aine. *Cah Med* 1982; **7**(20): 1205–1218.

23 Stoppa R, Petit J, Abourachid H. Procède original de plastie des hernies de l'aine: L'interposition sans fixation d'une prosthese en tulle de Dacron par voie mediane sous-peritoneale. *Chirurgie* 1973; **99**: 119–123.

24 Stoppa R, Petit J, Henry X. Unsaturated Dacron prosthesis in groin hernias. *Int Surg* 1975; **60**(8): 411–412.

25 Stoppa R, Henry X, Verhaeghe P. Place des prostheses reticulées non resorbables dans le traitement chirurgical des hernies de l'aine. *Chirurgie* 1981; **107**(5): 333–341.

26 Stoppa R, Henry X, Verhaeghe P. Place des prostheses dans le traitement des hernies de l'aine. *Bordeaux Med* 1982; **15**: 243–250.

27 Stoppa R, Warlaumont C, Verhaeghe P. Properitoneal placement of Dacron mesh in the repair of groin hernias. *Surg Rounds* 1983; **6**(4): 38–51.

28 Stoppa RE, Rives JL, Worlaumont C. The use of Dacron in the repair of hernias of the groin. *Surg Clin North Am* 1984; **64**: 269–286.

29 Stoppa RE, Warlaumont CR, Verhaeghe PJ, Romera ER, M'Balla-N'Di CJ. Prosthetic repair in the treatment of groin hernias. *Int Surg* 1986; **71**: 154–158.

Chapter 4
Endoscopic view of the anatomy of the inguinal region

P.A. Paraskeva, A. Darzi and J.R.T. Monson

The successful repair of an inguinal hernia relies on sound anatomical knowledge regardless of the technique used. This fact is well demonstrated by the laparoscopic hernia repair. The anatomy of the inguinal region as viewed from inside the abdomen is a new perspective and tends to be unfamiliar to surgeons who are accustomed to the anterior orientation of open hernia repair. Furthermore, structures that are visible from the anterior approach, such as the inguinal ligament and pubic tubercle, cannot easily be seen laparoscopically. Conversely, structures that would usually require extensive dissection with an open approach, such as the iliopubic tract and Cooper's ligament, can easily be viewed through the laparoscope.

Orientation in the inguinal region

Figure 4.1 shows the view obtained by the surgeon during laparoscopic hernia repair and illustrates important structures for orientation in the inguinal region. Orientation in the inguinal region after placing a laparoscope into the abdomen can be achieved by the identification of four key anatomical landmarks. These landmarks are the inferior epigastric vessels, the medial umbilical ligament, the

Figure 4.1

IE, inferior epigastric vessels; IR, internal inguinal ring; MUL, medial umbilical ligament; VD, vas deferens; EIV, external iliac vessels; GV, gonadal vessels.

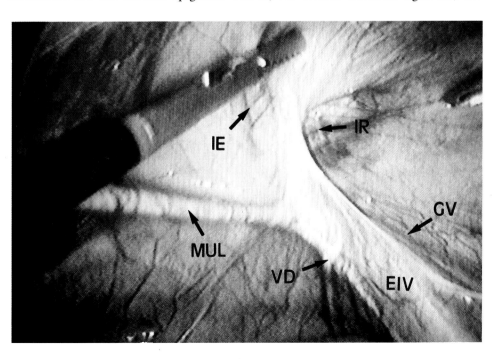

gonadal vessels and the vas deferens in the male and the round ligament of the uterus in the female.

Anatomy of the inguinal region

On entering the peritoneal cavity the most prominent structure encountered is the medial umbilical ligament. This is the remnant of the umbilical artery and can be seen in the superior field of view as a thick cord-like structure with an apparent mesentery running towards the umbilicus. Lying lateral to the medial umbilical ligament are the inferior epigastric vessels (Fig. 4.2). These vessels are most apparent medial to the internal inguinal ring and can be seen running superiorly and medially deep to the transversalis fascia which they then pierce to enter the rectus sheath. The inferior epigastric vessels are easily visualized in the thinner patient, and can often be seen pulsating. In the obese patient the layer of preperitoneal fat is thicker and the inferior epigastric vessels may be more difficult to find.

Lying lateral to the inferior epigastric vessels is the internal inguinal ring (Fig. 4.2). This may be a difficult structure to identify in the normal patient as it often only

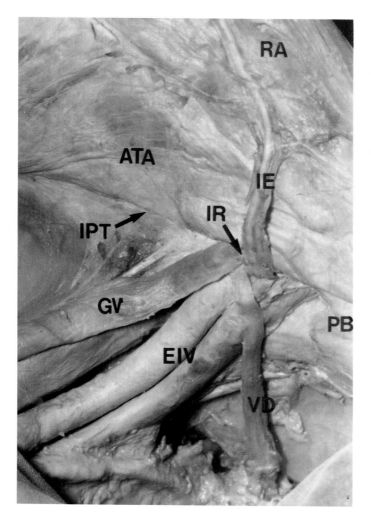

Figure 4.2
RA, rectus abdominus; ATA, arching fibres of transversus abdominus; IPT, iliopubic tract; IR, internal inguinal ring; IE, inferior epigastric vessels; GV, gonadal vessels; EIV, external iliac vessels; VD, vas deferens; PB, pubic bone.

appears as a dimple in the peritoneum. The internal ring is easier to identify in patients with indirect inguinal hernias as the internal ring is dilated and the defect can be visualized. Accurate location of the internal ring is achieved by finding the point of convergence of the gonadal vessels and the vas deferens or the round ligament.

The gonadal vessel can be seen as flat structures that traverse from lateral to medial in the inguinal region (Fig. 4.2). Since these structures are covered only by a layer of peritoneum, they are easily visualized. The gonadal vessels enter the internal ring at which point in the male they are joined by the vas deferens. The vas deferens can be seen as a cord-like structure travelling from medial lateral toward the internal inguinal ring (Fig. 4.2). The vas deferens is adherent to the layer of peritoneum covering it and is always associated with the artery to the vas which may aid in its visualization. The spermatic cord is formed at the posterior aspect of the internal inguinal ring.

As the gonadal vessels and the vas deferens merge to enter the inguinal canal, they form the apex of an imaginary triangle in the inguinal region. This has been termed the 'triangle of doom' by Spaw et al. [1], but unlike other anatomical triangles, such as the femoral triangle, this only has two sides. Therefore this area would be more accurately described as an 'angle of doom' [2]. The importance of recognizing this area when repairing a hernia laparoscopically is that between the gonadal vessels and the vas deferens, deep to the peritoneum lie the external iliac artery and vein (Fig. 4.2). To avoid damage to these vessels, extreme care must be taken when dissecting peritoneal flaps around this area. Also suturing and stapling should be restricted to medial and lateral to this area. However, stapling too far lateral could lead to damage of the lateral cutaneous nerve of the thigh which runs posterolateral to the caecum on the right and posterior to the descending colon on the left before passing behind or through the inguinal ligament. Damage to the lateral cutaneous nerve can lead to the patient experiencing postoperative paraesthesia or pain over the lateral aspect of the thigh [3]. The recognition that the area 3–4 cm lateral to the internal ring also contains vital structures has led to the angle of doom's margins being extended to form a 'quadrant of doom'.

The view of the anatomy described can be obscured on the left due to the position of the colon. This is because the preperitoneal reflection from the left paracolic gutter and sigmoid mesentery commonly obscures the view of the gonadal vessels and the vas deferens on the left side, and may also be included in the sac of the hernia. Care must therefore be taken when dissecting in this area during a left inguinal hernia repair.

A superficial incision in the peritoneum will reveal the anatomy of the inguinal region in greater detail. It exposes the preperitoneal fascia which envelopes the cord structures and contains a variable amount of fat. Dissection of peritoneal flaps should be done with care as the vas deferens and the gonadal vessels are adherent to the overlying peritoneum.

After complete dissection of the preperitoneal space, an exceptional posterior view of the anatomy of the anterior abdominal wall is obtained. Careful examination of this area reveals structures likely to be used in repair such as the iliopubic tract, Cooper's ligament and the arching fibres of the transversus abdominus muscle

(Fig. 4.2). Accurate identification of these aponeuroticofascial margins of the internal inguinal ring is important regardless of the type of laparoscopic repair.

The iliopubic tract is an important anatomical structure in laparoscopic hernia repair and was described in great detail by Nyhus [4]. It is a condensation of transversalis fascia and the most inferior part of the transversus abdominus aponeurosis. It begins laterally along the crest of the ilium from the anterior superior spine. The iliopubic tract then arches over the psoas muscle and the femoral vessels where it forms an integral part of the anterior femoral sheath. It continues medially to mark the inferior border of the internal inguinal ring before inserting on the superior pubic ramus, just lateral to Cooper's ligament. The most inferior fibres recurve into the normal groin which forms the medial border of the femoral canal. The iliopubic tract is distinct from the inguinal ligament, but serves as an important landmark for this structure which is superficial to it.

Cooper's ligament is a thick condensation of transversalis fascia and periosteum over the superior pubic ramus. The course of this ligament is curvilinear, proceeding medially to form the prominence of the pelvic brim anteriorly. Careful dissection is required to uncover this structure which appears glossy white. It is important to identify Cooper's ligament and the iliopubic tract as these provide secure sites for the anchoring of a prosthetic mesh.

The arching fibres of transversus abdominus can be seen travelling over the internal ring and Hesselbach's triangle to insert medially onto the pubis anterior to the rectus abdominus muscle.

When performing a laparoscopic hernia repair it is important to identify the type of hernia. The type of hernia can be identified by its relationship to the inferior epigastric vessels (Fig. 4.3). A direct inguinal hernia will be medial to the inferior

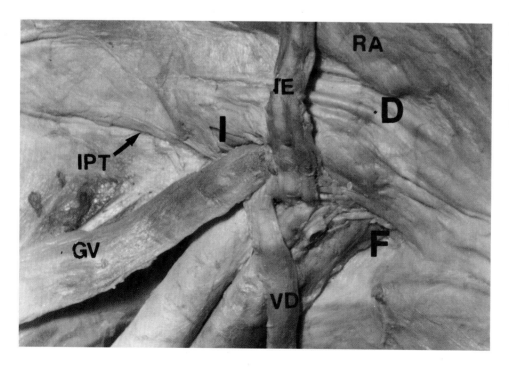

Figure 4.3
RA, rectus abdominus; IE, inferior epigastric vessels; IPT, iliopubic tract; GV, gonadal vessels; VD, vas deferens; I, indirect; D, direct; F, femoral.

epigastric vessels, in Hesselbach's triangle. An indirect inguinal hernia will be seen as a dilatation of the internal inguinal ring and will therefore be lateral to the inferior epigastric vessels. A femoral hernia will pass through the femoral canal and therefore inferior to the iliopubic tract, medial to the inferior epigastric vessels and lateral to Cooper's ligament.

Insertion and positioning of the mesh

Having established the anatomy of the inguinal region from the point of view of safe laparoscopic dissection and identified the key landmarks to which the prosthetic mesh will be stapled, the mesh is inserted and positioned. The mesh must be large enough to cover all potential hernia sites in the inguinal region. The inferomedial corner of the mesh is secured to Cooper's ligament; the medial border of the mesh overlaps the lateral border of the rectus abdominus muscle to which it is stapled. The superior border of the mesh is stapled to the arching fibres of transversus abdominus. No staples are placed below the iliopubic tract (Fig. 4.4). Not placing staples below the iliopubic tract limits the chance of damaging important structures that are found in this area and also decreases the incidence of postoperative neuralgias following damage to important nerves such as the lateral cutaneous nerve of the thigh.

Figure 4.4
ATA, arching fibres of transversus abdominus; IE, inferior epigastric vessels; RA, rectus abdominus; IR, internal inguinal ring; IPT, iliopubic tract; GV, gonadal vessels; EIV, external iliac vessels; VD, vas deferens; CL, Cooper's ligament.

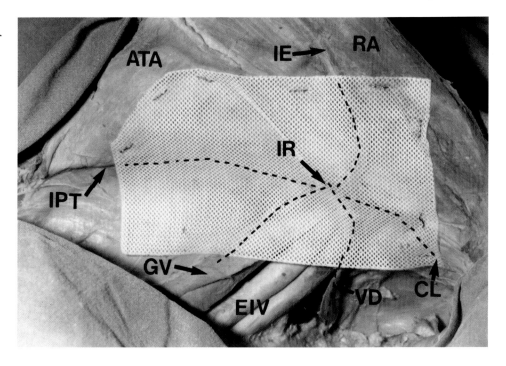

The positioning of the prosthetic mesh in the fashion described adequately covers the direct, indirect and femoral hernia sites (Fig. 4.5). This thereby decreases the chance of postoperative recurrence in any of these areas.

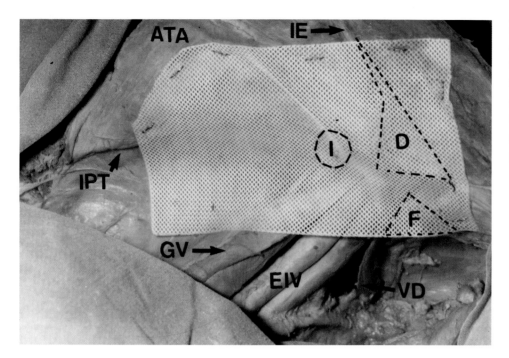

Figure 4.5

ATA, arching fibres of transversus abdominus; IE, inferior epigastric vessels; IPT, iliopubic tract; GV, gonadal vessels; EIV, external iliac vessels; VD, vas deferens; I, indirect; D, direct; F, femoral.

Conclusion

A precise and thorough knowledge of the anatomical relationships in the inguinal region is perhaps the single most important determinant of complication-free laparoscopic hernia repair. Although novice laparoscopists initially may find anatomical orientation difficult, accurate identification of key structures and landmarks is essential and can help promote safe and practical methods for laparoscopic inguinal hernia repair.

References

1 Spaw AT, Ennis BW, Spaw LP. Laparoscopic hernia repair: the anatomical basis. *J Laparoendosc Surg* 1991; **1**: 269–277.
2 Paraskeva PA, Darzi A, Guillou PJ, Monson JRT. An endoscopic view of the surgical anatomy of the inguinal region. *Min Invas Ther* 1993; **2**: 313–318.
3 MacFadyen BV, Corbitt J, Spaw AT. Complications of laparoscopic herniorrhaphy. *Surg Endosc* 1993; **7**: 155–158.
4 Nyhus LM, Condon RE (eds). *Hernia*. JB Lippincott, Philadelphia, 1989: 18–64.

Chapter 5

Introduction to laparoscopic hernia repair and review of published data

P.A. Paraskeva, J.R.T. Monson and A. Darzi

Few recent developments in surgery have earned such widespread acclaim as therapeutic laparoscopy. These minimal access techniques have changed the approach to many surgical procedures and promise to change many more. One such procedure is laparoscopic inguinal hernia repair, which is receiving widespread interest from many general surgeons. Although many are excited by laparoscopic hernia repair, surgeons have been very cautious in accepting the laparoscopic approach as the open hernia repair does not violate the peritoneal cavity and can be carried out under local anaesthetic on an outpatient basis [1, 2].

Inguinal hernia is the second most commonly treated general surgical condition, accounting for 15% of operating time annually, and debate continues regarding its aetiology and optimal management [3–5]. Although open hernia repair performed under local anaesthetic remains the standard, disability, recurrence rates and complications such as infection, groin haematoma, ilioinguinal nerve entrapment and ischaemic orchitis remain perplexing problems [3]. Additionally, recovery from open hernia repair can often be painful and prolonged and return to normal activity may take up to 6–8 weeks.

Laparoscopic hernia repair is an evolving procedure and offers new opportunities for groin hernia repair. Laparoscopy has been proposed as a logical surgical approach because, firstly, it offers the most direct access to the posterior inguinal wall and, secondly, if a mesh is used the repair will be tension free. The importance of removing tension from a hernia repair was proposed by Lichtenstein [4]. Lichtenstein felt the prime cause for hernia recurrence was the suturing together of structures not normally in apposition causing a distortion of the normal anatomy and suture line tension. He subsequently proposed the 'tension-free hernioplasty', an anterior hernia repair in which a polypropylene mesh is used to strengthen the posterior inguinal wall [5]. This technique has enjoyed good results so far [1]. The laparoscopic mesh repairs therefore apply the same surgical principles except the mesh is placed from the inside.

The laparoscopic hernia repair was proposed by Ger in 1982, after he described a series of patients in which inguinal hernias were managed through a transabdominal approach. The hernias were repaired at routine laparotomy for other conditions [6]. Ger closed the hernial orifice without dissection, ligation or reduction of the sac using steel clips. He noted only one recurrence in a series of 13 patients with a follow-up of 44 months. In one of the patients in this series, Ger applied staples to close the hernial defect under laparoscopic guidance. This patient was followed up for 8 years without evidence of recurrence, and this represents the first laparoscopic hernia repair in humans. Ger and colleagues devised a stapling instrument (the 'herniostat') for endoscopic closure of the neck of the indirect hernial sac and evaluated it in dogs [7]. The results showed the sac to be obliterated in five animals and significantly reduced in another eight. These results together with the prototype laparoscopic hernia stapler prompted Ger to propose laparoscopic hernia repair as an advantageous method for managing hernia.

The concept of the laparoscopic hernia repair itself was first presented by Bogjavalenski at the 18th meeting of the American Association of Gynaecological Laparoscopists in 1989. He described a procedure that involved the introduction of a rolled piece of polypropylene mesh placed in the indirect hernial sac. In 1990 Schultz *et al.* used a similar technique of filling the hernial defect with pieces of polypropylene mesh and then closing the peritoneum over it. This group published data on the first series of patients. Unfortunately their early results showed a high recurrence rate [8]. After this, Schultz modified his technique by stapling a flat piece of mesh over the plugged hernial defect which yielded better results.

From these early beginnings many different methods of laparoscopic hernia repair have evolved. However, all authors subscribe to the idea that laparoscopic hernia repair offers many potential benefits. These benefits include smaller wounds, a reduced chance of injury to the spermatic cord and the testis, an avoidance of ilioinguinal postoperative neuralgias, and the ability to diagnose and treat bilateral inguinal hernias without extensive dissection. These potential advantages plus the hope that laparoscopic hernia repair will yield lower recurrence rates and earlier return to work have given surgeons the incentive to refine their techniques.

Despite modifications in technique a common problem remains. The anatomy of the inguinal region encountered through the laparoscope is presented in a different perspective to that usually seen in the standard anterior approach. Sound knowledge of the endoscopic anatomy of the inguinal region is necessary if the hernia is to be repaired safely and effectively (see Chapter 4).

Methods of laparoscopic hernia repair

Ring closure techniques (RC)

The ring closure initially championed by Ger [7] is an uncomplicated technique which consists of a high ligation of the indirect hernia sac and closure of the internal ring using clips or suture. The ring closure technique is a logical approach in young patients and patients with small indirect inguinal hernias.

The lateral suture ring closure technique as advocated by Spaw [9] can be used to repair minimally dilated rings. In this technique the peritoneum is dissected to reveal the transversus abdominus arch. This is sutured, using continuous or interrupted non-absorbable suture, to Cooper's ligament or the iliopubic tract. This repair is similar to the open preperitoneal iliopubic tract technique used by Nyhus [10]. The transversus abdominus arch is approximated to the iliopubic tract which closes the internal inguinal ring. This type of repair is not recommended for large indirect, direct or femoral hernias.

A modification of the lateral suture repair was described by Gazayerli [11]. This procedure involved approximating the transversus abdominus arch and the iliopubic tract. In the original description of the procedure Gazayerli placed mesh in the defect prior to the iliopubic tract repair. Subsequently this technique has been modified and a mesh is now placed in the preperitoneal space after the iliopubic tract repair.

More recently a technique has been described by Geraghty *et al.* [12] in which a sutured repair of the internal inguinal ring using a hollow J-needle is introduced percutaneously just lateral to the inferior epigastric vessels.

The plug and mesh repair (P and M)

The plugging of femoral hernias and small recurrent hernias has been used during open hernia repair [13]. The laparoscopic plugging of the hernial defect was proposed by Schultz [8] and developed by Corbitt [14] and was based on the anterior plug repairs. The laparoscopic repair consisted of incising the peritoneum of the hernial defect and then stuffing small pieces of polypropylene mesh into the defect. This was thought to eliminate the space with scarring helping to decrease the space further. The high recurrence rate associated with this procedure has led to its fall from favour despite modifications made to it by Schultz [15].

The extraperitoneal mesh technique (EPMR)

The extraperitoneal repair was developed by McKernan and Laws [16]. This technique is an endoscopically guided hernia repair performed without entering the peritoneal cavity. It is therefore not truly a laparoscopic procedure, as this implies entry into the peritoneal cavity. Instead the laparoscopic instruments are manipulated in a working space outside the peritoneal cavity, in the extraperitoneal space. In the procedure the dissecting instruments are used to free the peritoneum from the overlying rectus abdominus muscle. This dissection develops a preperitoneal tunnel for the placement of additional instruments. The peritoneum is dissected down to the pubic bone and Cooper's ligament; the hernial sac can then be visualized. The defect is then covered with polypropylene mesh, which is stapled into place using Cooper's ligament, the iliopubic tract and the rectus abdominus as anchoring sites.

Transabdominal preperitoneal repair (TAPP)

This is perhaps the most commonly performed approach. Arregui *et al.* [17] first described a repair using a mesh placed preperitoneally. The peritoneum is incised in a horizontal line above the defect. Two flaps are then fashioned by dissecting the peritoneum away from the transversalis fascia, Cooper's ligament, vas and gonadal vessels. A polypropylene mesh is then cut to approximately 10×12 cm to cover the direct, indirect and femoral hernia areas. This mesh is then stapled into place using

Cooper's ligament, the iliopubic tract, transversus abduminus and the lateral border of the rectus as anchoring sites. The peritoneal flaps are then stapled together over the mesh to prevent bowel adhesion to the mesh.

This method is ideal for repairing bilateral inguinal hernias as the dissection may be continued horizontally from one inguinal region to the other. For bilateral repair, a single large piece of mesh is used and stapled as before.

The intraperitoneal onlay patch repair (IPOM)

In this repair the prosthetic mesh is placed transperitoneally on top of the peritoneum as advocated by Toy and Smoot [18] and Salerno et al. [19]. This approach is attractive for many reasons. Firstly, it is simple and speedy to carry out since the path is simply stapled over the hernial defect. Secondly, no peritoneal dissection is required which also contributes to less postoperative pain together with the potential for this to be carried out under local anaesthetic.

The major concern with this technique is the placement of an exposed mesh in the abdominal cavity. This raises anxiety about bowel adhesions to the mesh and possible fistula formation. Alternative meshes have been used in these repairs, such as expanded polytetrafluoroethylene (PTFE). However, one problem is that repairs performed with these meshes are dependent on the strength of the mesh only, because of the minimal fibrous ingrowth. Early results have been encouraging but careful follow-up of these patients is required together with the development of safer mesh repairs.

Evaluation of laparoscopic inguinal hernia and its complications

Due to the relatively recent introduction of laparoscopic hernia repair the data that exist on the effectiveness of these techniques are limited. The follow-up is short and consequently it is difficult to draw solid conclusions. Despite this, authors have published their initial experiences with laparoscopic hernia repair of varying techniques. Table 5.1 shows the types of hernias repaired by varying techniques by different authors.

Table 5.1

Results and follow-up length of some major laparoscopic hernia series, of varying techniques.

Series	Type	No. of hernias/ no. of recurrences	Max. follow-up (months)
Darzi et al. [20]	TAPP	155/2	18
McKernan and Laws [16]	EPMR	54/0	12
Ger et al. [7]	Suture	27/1	64
Arregui et al. [17]	TAPP	94/1	28
Corbitt [14]	Plug	35/3	15
Schultz et al. [8]	Plug	198/8	24
MacFadyen et al. [23]	IPOM	102/2	13

One of the largest coordinated multicentred trials was described by MacFadyen *et al.* [23] in the United States. This study involved 79 surgeons repairing 841 inguinal hernias in 762 patients. During this study six variations on the laparoscopic hernia repair were evaluated. Type 1 repair was a sutured ring closure; the follow-up on these patients was 24 months and during this period it was noted that 2.2% of patients presented with testicular pain, which was the only minor complication. The recurrence rate was 2.2%. The type 2 repair was a plug and mesh repair which was followed up for 8 months. There was a 6.8% recurrence rate, 3.4% were able to palpate the mesh in the inguinal region, and in one patient the mesh actually migrated down to the scrotum. Additionally, there was one incidence of bladder injury and a 1.1% incidence of hydroceles. The high rate of complications associated with this technique prompted the authors to discontinue this procedure.

They also evaluated three types of laparoscopic stapled mesh repairs. The first of these was the intraperitoneal onlay patch repair which involved 186 hernia repairs followed for 5 months. There was a 3.2% recurrence rate with this technique, three patients sustained bladder injuries, two developed hydroceles, one patient developed pain over the lateral aspect of the thigh and there was one instance of pubic osteitis. Many of these complications resolved after a 3-week period.

The second type of mesh repair was the transabdominal preperitoneal patch repair which involved the largest number of reported repairs. The patients were followed for an average of 5 months and during this time there was a 0.8% recurrence rate. Minor complications included scrotal haematomas in 3%, pain over the lateral aspect of the thigh in 2.2%, while urinary retention was observed in 2% of patients. The numbness of the thigh resolved in all patients after 3–4 weeks.

The final type of mesh repair evaluated was the extraperitoneal hernia repair. These patients were followed up for 7 months and no recurrences were noted. Haematomas developed in 6%, and 1.1% experienced testicular pain. All the minor complications of this technique resolved after 3 weeks on conservative management.

Other groups have published results on laparoscopic hernia repair, many of them on the transabdominal preperitoneal patch repair. Both Seid *et al.* [21] and Newman *et al.* [22] reported results using the preperitoneal mesh repair. Seid *et al.* reported on 27 patients; they encountered no recurrences within a 7-month follow-up. Newman *et al.* repaired 102 hernias with 1% recurrence rate and found this repair to be safe and effective. In the United Kingdom our own group investigated our first 126 transabdominal preperitoneal mesh repairs [20]. We experienced three recurrences with a mean follow-up of 18 months. There were also minor complications such as hydroceles in two patients, scrotal haematomas in six patients, and pain over the lateral aspect of the thigh in another two patients. All these minor symptoms settled on conservative management. The most serious complication to date was an incomplete bowel obstruction due to herniation of a section of small bowel between the staples in the peritoneum; this led to death from an aspiration pneumonia. Bowel obstruction following a transabdominal preperitoneal repair has been reported before by Hendrickse and Evans [24] and is increasingly being recognized as a pitfall with the approach. Overall the worldwide incidence averages 1% and this has led many groups to further evaluate the extraperitoneal approach where the peritoneal surface is not violated.

Discussion

Following the success of laparoscopic cholecystectomy [25–28], surgeons have examined other areas of abdominal and thoracic surgery for possible endoscopic applications. Inguinal hernia repair is one of the most common general surgical procedures [22], but despite many developments in traditional open methods of hernia repair there continues to be a significant incidence of complications [3]. The potential advantages of laparoscopic repair to the patient in terms of reduced disability and decreased groin discomfort made the treatment of inguinal hernia an attractive proposition.

Laparoscopic hernia repair is a rapidly evolving procedure. Just as there are many traditional ways to repair a hernia, many different techniques have been reported for laparoscopic hernia repair.

The laparoscopic hernia repair raises many discussion points. Firstly, undertaking a laparoscopic hernia repair requires different technical considerations to the standard open approaches.

Many surgeons have not welcomed laparoscopic hernia repair with open arms. This reluctance has primarily been due to the fact that at present a general anaesthetic is required to perform a laparoscopic repair, the long-term results are unproven and the potential for further operative complications seems extensive. Many find this unacceptable when standard anterior hernia repairs can be successfully performed using local anaesthetic [1, 2]. Although many centres have used local anaesthesia for diagnostic laparoscopy, the greater pneumoperitoneum, together with peritoneal dissection required in some techniques, has made local anaesthesia unsuitable for laparoscopic hernia repair at present. Some techniques such as the onlay patch repair do offer the potential to be performed under local anaesthesia as there is no peritoneal dissection involved, but until the repair is shown to be efficacious this potential may not be realized.

Another technical consideration of the laparoscopic hernia repair concerns the use of mesh. Meshes are commonly used in laparoscopic hernia repairs such as the plug and mesh repair, onlay patch repair, preperitoneal repair and the extraperitoneal repair. Surgeons generally have been reluctant to use prosthetic material when repairing a hernia due to the increased risk of infection. A variety of materials have been used over the years for hernia repair such as autogenous (e.g. fascia lata) or more inert materials such as polypropylene (Marlex) or Dacron (Mersilene) [30, 31]. These are incorporated by the host's fibroblasts during organization of wound healing. The use of mesh has been advocated in an open preperitoneal repair by Stoppa *et al.* [31] and more recently by Lichtenstein in the tension-free hernioplasty—an anterior hernia repair [5].

Lichtenstein's results suggest that using a mesh is safe and durable and therefore justify their use laparoscopically. The use of a mesh to repair the posterior inguinal wall during a laparoscopic preperitoneal repair is the same as a Lichtenstein repair except that the mesh is placed behind the defect instead of anteriorly.

During the evolution of the laparoscopic mesh repair the size of the mesh used by surgeons has changed. Initially surgeons tailored meshes to cover only the hernial defect. However, now the feeling is that to reduce the risk of recurrence a larger mesh should be used. Stoppa *et al.* [31] felt that the medial aspect of Hesselbach's triangle and the area immediately superior to the femoral vessels were the most likely regions for recurrence. To cover these areas the mesh must be 12×10 cm or larger. We have also found it important to use a large mesh that covers the direct hernia site, i.e. Hesselbach's triangle, the indirect hernia site and the femoral hernia site [20]. This, we presume, will decrease the risk of recurrence still further.

It has also been found that fixation of the mesh is important whether staples or the more difficult and time-consuming sutures are used. The mesh plugging techniques used by Schultz *et al.* [8] and Corbitt [14] showed unacceptable recurrence rates and incidences of mesh migration. Adequate fixation of the mesh to structures such as the pubic bone, Cooper's ligament and the transversus abdominus is particularly important. If this is not done the mesh may bulge into the defect or mesh migration may occur. New types of staples have been developed that anchor the mesh more securely when stapled to these structures.

Another major area for discussion has been the management of the hernia sac. Ger simply closed the internal inguinal ring and left the sac in place thereby reducing the damage to cord structures caused by dissection. Others have dissected the sac but have noted an increased incidence of testicular pain and haematoma. Salerno *et al.* [19] recommended leaving the sac in place and circumcising it at the neck, before placing a mesh over the defect. Other surgeons, such as Corbitt [14], have amputated the sac using a linear laparoscopic stapler, whereas McKernan ligated the sac and removed it during an extraperitoneal repair. It does seem likely that dissection of the sac causes an increased incidence of haematoma and scrotal pain postoperatively. In our patients we no longer dissect the sac as we also felt this was the prime cause of scrotal haematoma. We also advocate leaving the sac in place, or circumcising it at its neck, and have not encountered any problem associated with leaving the hernial sac. It seems that leaving the hernial sac in place does not create any problems or affect the integrity of the repair in any way.

A common problem encountered after laparoscopic hernia repair has been numbness or paraesthesia over the lateral aspect of the thigh which is a recognized complication [32]. This is most likely to be due to irritation of the lateral femoral cutaneous nerve. This may have developed during dissection or the placement of staples. The nerve itself is not easily visualized laparoscopically, therefore accurate anatomical knowledge of its path of travel is required to avoid dissecting or stapling in the area near it. This problem though has been found to settle down 4–6 weeks after the operation on non-steroidal anti-inflammatory drugs.

A complication that has begun to cause concern is the incidence of small bowel obstruction that occurs following a transabdominal preperitoneal mesh repair due to herniation of small bowel between staples in the peritoneum [24]. Therefore, maybe a shift to the use of techniques such as the extraperitoneal repair, where the peritoneum is not incised, may lead to more favourable results and decrease the incidence of this dangerous complication.

Together with the complications specific to the laparoscopic inguinal hernia repair, the complications of laparoscopy in general must be considered. Firstly, this laparoscopic procedure must be carried out under a general anaesthetic, which carries with it its own problems. Also there are complications associated with production of a pneumoperitoneum such as shoulder tip pain and subcutaneous emphysema. Other complications associated with laparoscopy are the increased risk, albeit small, of visceral damage and damage to major vessels. The need for the use of endoscopic diathermy also carries with it the risk of intra-abdominal burn injuries [33].

These problems together with the learning curve that needs to be overcome in using laparoscopic equipment and developing adequate hand–eye coordination may discourage some surgeons. Therefore, how can a laparoscopic approach be justified? The logic behind a laparoscopic approach to inguinal hernia can be explained from many perspectives. Firstly, anatomically: restoring the integrity of the posterior inguinal wall is fundamental in repairing a hernia. Laparoscopy gives the most direct access to the posterior inguinal wall, unlike the standard anterior approach which requires much more tissue dissection to reveal this structure. Another justification for laparoscopic hernia repair is that if a mesh repair is employed the repair will be tension free, and will therefore be like a Lichtenstein repair [5] except that the mesh is placed posteriorly.

Secondly, from the patient's point of view laparoscopy offers many potential benefits. Laparoscopy potentially eliminates the complications of standard hernia repair such as wound haematoma and infection, ischaemic orchitis and damage to the ilioinguinal nerve and the spermatic cord [3]. The smaller abdominal wounds also lead to less postoperative pain. The major desire of surgeons is to decrease the recurrence rate of inguinal hernia repair and shorten the time taken to return to work. At the moment it is too early to say with confidence that the recurrence rate using a laparoscopic approach is better than for open repairs as a longer follow-up is required. Thus far, studies have shown that after a laparoscopic repair patients return to work within 10 days postoperatively [17, 22]. This compares favourably with the time taken to return to work for an anterior hernia repair done under local anaesthesia [1].

The reduction of patient discomfort and the early return to work has economic implications for the health service and for industry in general. Centres that undertake laparoscopy do so with the hope of reduction of postoperative discomfort for the patient and earlier return to work. Laparoscopic hernia repair is a more costly procedure than a standard open hernia repair because of the use of specialist disposable laparoscopic instruments, for example the hernia stapler. The market for specialist laparoscopic tools has been exploited by equipment manufacturers who have discovered a lucrative niche for the development of these tools.

The laparoscopic hernia repair is a relatively new procedure and as with all new procedures there is a learning curve to overcome. In an effort to ensure the safety of the patient and promote high standards in laparoscopic surgery, the Royal College of Surgeons of England have laid down guidelines for surgeons [34]. As a consequence of this, together with the increased interest in laparoscopy, various centres have established laparoscopic hernia teaching courses where surgeons are guided through the procedure by surgeons already proficient in the technique.

Summary

Inguinal hernia repair is one of the most common general surgical conditions. The results from conventional hernia repairs have been far from satisfactory. This fact plus the exciting possibilities offered by laparoscopy has led to the development of laparoscopic hernia repair techniques. The laparoscopic inguinal hernia repair offers an attractive alternative to the conventional open approach if it can be shown to be efficacious.

The potential benefits offered by the laparoscopic hernia repair must be confirmed by data addressing important issues such as long-term recurrence rates and postoperative complications. Until such time, no cast iron assumptions about this approach can be made. Many different laparoscopic hernia techniques exist but no one technique has been shown to be superior. A large, randomized control study is required comparing the laparoscopic repair with an open approach; surgeons will then be in a more favourable position to judge whether laparoscopic hernia repair offers an advantageous approach or not.

Laparoscopic hernia repair is in an evolving state but early experiences show that this approach is technically feasible and relatively safe. The advantages associated with repairing an inguinal hernia laparoscopically must be proved beyond doubt if this procedure is to earn a regular place in general surgical practice.

References

1 Shulman AG, Amid PK, Lichtenstein IL. The safety of mesh repair for primary inguinal hernia—results of 3019 operations from five diverse sources. *Am Surg* 1992; **58**: 255–257.

2 Glasgow F. Short stay surgery (Shouldice technique) for repair of inguinal hernia. *Ann R Coll Surg Engl* 1984; **66**: 382–387.

3 Wantz GE. Complications of inguinal hernia repair. *Surg Clin North Am* 1984; **64**: 287–298.

4 Lichtenstein IL, Shulman AG, Amid PK *et al*. The pathophysiology of recurrent hernia introducing a new concept of the tension free repair. *Contemp Surg* 1989; **35**: 13–18.

5 Lichtenstein IL, Shulman AG, Amid PK *et al*. The tension free hernioplasty. *Am J Surg* 1989; **157**: 188–192.

6 Ger R. The management of certain abdominal hernias by intra-abdominal closure of the sac. *Ann R Coll Surg Engl* 1982; **64**: 342.

7 Ger R, Monroe K, Duvivier R *et al*. Management of indirect inguinal hernias by laparoscopic closure of the neck of the sac. *Am J Surg* 1990; **159**: 370.

8 Schultz L, Graber J, Pietrafitta J *et al*. Laser laparoscopic herniorrhapy: A clinical trial: Preliminary results. *J Laparoendosc Surg* 1990; **1**: 41.

9 Spaw AT, Ennis BW, Spaw LP. Laparoscopic hernia repair: the anatomic basis. *J Laparoendosc Surg* 1991; **1**: 269–277.

10 Nyhus LM, Condon RE (eds). *Hernia*, 3rd edn. JB Lippincott, Philadelphia, 1989: 3–17

11 Gazayerli MM. Anatomical laparoscopic hernia repair of direct or indirect inguinal hernias using the transversalis fascia and the iliopubic tract. *Surg Laparosc Endosc* 1992; **2**: 49–52.

12 Geraghty JG, Grace PA, Quereshi A, Bouchier-Hayes D, Osborne DH. Simple new technique for laparoscopic inguinal hernia repair. *Br J Surg* 1994; **81**: 93.

13 Robbins AW, Rutkow IM. The mesh-plug hernioplasty. *Surg Clin North Am* **1993; 73**: 501–511.

14 Corbitt JD. Laparoscopic herniorrhaphy. *Surg Laparosc Endosc* 1991; **1**: 23.

15 Corbitt JD. Transabdominal preperitoneal herniorrhaphy. *Surg Laparosc Endosc* 1993; **4**: 328–332.

16 McKernan BJ, Laws HL. Laparoscopic repair of inguinal hernias using a totally extraperitoneal prosthetic approach. *Surg Endosc* 1993; **7**: 26–28.

17 Arregui M, Davis C, Yucel O, Nagan R. Laparoscopic mesh repair of inguinal hernia using a preperitoneal approach: A preliminary report. *Surg Laparosc Endosc* 1992; **2**(1): 53–58.

18 Toy FK, Smoot RT Jr. Toy–Smoot laparoscopic hernioplasty. *Surg Laparosc Endosc* 1991; **1**: 151.

19 Salerno GM, Fitzgibbons RJ Jr, Hart RO *et al*. Laparoscopic herniorrhaphy. In Zucker KA (ed.) *Surgical Laparoscopic Update 1*. Quality Medical Publishing, Inc., St Louis, 1992.

20 Darzi A, Paraskeva PA, Quereshi A, Menzies-Gow N, Guillou PJ, Monson JRT. Laparoscopic herniorrhaphy: Initial experience in 126 cases. *J Laparoendosc Surg* 1994 (In press).

21 Seid AS, Deutsch H, Jacobson A. Laparoscopic herniorrhaphy. *Surg Laparosc Endosc* 1992; **2**: 59–60.

22 Newman L, Eubanks S, Mason E, Duncan TD. Is laparoscopic herniorrhaphy an effective alternative to open hernia repair? *J Laparoendosc Surg* 1993; **3**: 121–128.

23 MacFadyen BV, Spaw AT, Corbitt J *et al.* Complications of laparoscopic herniorrhaphy. *Surg Endosc* 1993; **7**: 155–158.

24 Hendrickse CW, Evans DS. Intestinal obstruction following laparoscopic inguinal hernia repair. *Br J Surg* 1993; **80**: 1432.

25 Cuschieri A, Dubois F, Mouiel J *et al.* The European experience with laparoscopic cholecystectomy. *Am J Surg* 1991; **161**: 385–387.

26 Ganey JB, Johnson PA, Prillman PE, McSwain GR. Cholecystectomy: clinical experience with a large series. *Am J Surg* 1986; **156**: 352–357.

27 McSherry CK. Cholecystectomy: The gold standard. *Am J Surg* 1989; **158**: 174–178.

28 Pickleman J, Gonzalez RP. The improving results of cholecystectomy. *Arch Surg* 1986; **121**: 930–934.

29 Rutkow IM. Surgical operations and manpower: can technical proficiency be maintained? In *Socioeconomics of Surgery*. CV Mosby, St Louis, 1989: 16–17.

30 Read RC, Barone GW, Hauer-Jensen M, Yoder G. Preperitoneal prosthetic mesh placement through the groin. *Surg Clin North Am* 1993; **73**(3): 545–555.

31 Stoppa RE, Rives JL, Warlaumont CR *et al.* The use of Dacron in the repair of hernias of the groin. *Surg Clin North Am* 1984; **64**: 269.

32 Kraus MA. Nerve injury during laparoscopic inguinal hernia repair. *Surg Laparosc Endosc* 1993; **4**: 342–345.

33 Ponsky J. Complications of laparoscopic cholecystectomy. *Am J Surg* 1991; **161**: 393–397.

34 *Minimal Access Surgery: Laparoscopic Cholecystectomy and Related Gastrointestinal Procedures.* Royal College of Surgeons of England, December 1990.

Chapter 6
Initial results in transabdominal preperitoneal repair

A. Darzi, P.A. Paraskeva and J.R.T. Monson

The last chapter on the history of the groin anatomy and operative repair of hernia defects has not been written.

(Nyhus and Bombeck [1])

Laparoscopic hernia repair is among the most controversial endoscopic procedures currently practised and has been the subject of intense discussion. Many of the initial series of laparoscopic hernia repair describe techniques that incorporate the stapling of a prosthetic polypropylene mesh over the hernial defect for repair. The transabdominal preperitoneal patch (TAPP) repair initially described by Arregui *et al.* [2] has been one of the more popular methods of laparoscopic hernia repair that has been reported in the literature [3, 4]. The TAPP repair is a laparoscopic stapled mesh repair in which a transabdominal approach to the posterior inguinal wall is used. The principles behind repairing a hernia using a TAPP repair are firstly to identify the anatomical landmarks of the inguinal region; once this is done the type of hernia present can be identified. The peritoneum is then incised superior to the hernial defect and peritoneal flaps are developed using blunt dissection. After an extensive dissection of the extraperitoneal space, the anatomical landmarks to which the mesh will be stapled are identified. The prosthetic mesh is then positioned correctly and stapled to the underlying anatomical landmarks. Finally, the peritoneal flaps are closed over the prosthetic mesh to prevent adherence of the bowel.

Many groups have reported their initial results using the TAPP repair [3, 4]. In this chapter we report on our initial experience using the TAPP repair in 126 patients. The aim of this study is to investigate whether laparoscopic hernia repair offers a safe and effective alternative to traditional open hernia repair.

Materials and methods

In this study inguinal hernias in 126 patients were repaired using the TAPP method. The male to female ratio was 116:10 and the mean age of the patients was 49.8 (17–76) years.

All patients were placed under general anaesthesia in a 15–30° Trendelenburg inclination and the pneumoperitoneum was produced in the standard fashion. A three-port laparoscopic approach was used [4]. The hernia sac was retracted out of the inguinal canal and the peritoneum above the defect was incised using endoscopic scissors. Small indirect hernia sacs were everted as part of the peritoneal flap, but larger sacs were left in place and circumcised at their necks. Two peritoneal flaps were then created and the posterior inguinal wall was exposed. A rectangular piece of polypropylene mesh (8 × 12 cm) was fashioned. The mesh was then pushed through a port and stapled to the posterior inguinal wall using an endoscopic stapler. The mesh was anchored to Cooper's ligament, the iliopubic tract, the arching fibres of transversus abdominus and the lateral border of the rectus abdominus muscle. Important structures such as the inferior epigastric vessels, the vas deferens, gonadal vessels and the external iliac vessels were identified and avoided. After placement of the mesh the peritoneal flaps were reopposed with staples. The operative site was inspected for haemostasis, the abdomen desufflated and the skin closed.

Results

To date 126 patients have undergone TAPP repairs for inguinal hernias. There were no intraoperative complications and only one procedure had to be converted to an open operation. Forty-six patients had direct inguinal hernias, 56 had indirect inguinal hernias, and 24 had both; of these, 21 hernias were recurrent. Fifty-one hernias were right sided, 46 were left sided, and 29 were bilaterals. The mean operative time was 53 (20–95) min for unilateral hernia repair and 70 (50–210) min for bilateral hernia repair.

Three patients presented with evidence of postoperative recurrence, one of which occurred 2 months after the repair. One of these patients had an emergency exploration of a wound which was thought to be an incarcerated recurrent hernia; this was in fact a haematoma and not a recurrence. No vascular injuries of cord damage were noted; however, two patients presented within 48 h of the operation with paraesthesia along the distribution of the lateral cutaneous nerve of the thigh. These patients were treated with non-steroidal anti-inflammatory drugs and their symptoms resolved within 2 weeks of the procedure. Another two patients presented postoperatively with hydroceles, all of which resolved on conservative management. In addition, scrotal haematomas were noted in six patients which again were treated conservatively. Incomplete small bowel obstruction has been the only major postoperative complication to date: a loop of small bowel herniated between two staples in the peritoneum. This patient subsequently died due to aspiration pneumonia following the small bowel obstruction.

The mean hospital stay was 1.2 (1–3) days, the mean return to unrestricted activity was 8 (3–12) days and the mean follow-up to date has been 7 (1–18) months.

Discussion

Following the success of laparoscopic cholecystectomy [5–8], surgeons have examined other areas of abdominal and thoracic surgery for possible endoscopic applications. Inguinal hernia repair is one of the most common general surgical procedures [9], but despite many developments in traditional open methods of hernia repair there continues to be a significant incidence of complications [10]. The potential advantages of laparoscopic repair to the patient in terms of reduced disability and decreased groin discomfort made the treatment of inguinal hernia an attractive proposition.

Laparoscopic hernia repair is a rapidly evolving procedure. Just as there are many traditional ways to repair a hernia many different techniques have been reported for laparoscopic hernia repair. Laparoscopic herniorrhaphy was first suggested by Ger *et al.* after observing that intra-abdominal repair of hernia found during laparotomy for other procedures was effective [11]. Intra-abdominal repair was accomplished by closure of the internal hernial opening with clips or sutures.

In 1990 Schultz *et al.* [12] reported success with a mesh stuffing technique called the 'plug and mesh repair'. Corbitt later modified the technique by using a high ligation of the sac [13]. Both variations on this type of laparoscopic repair involved placing plugs of polypropylene mesh through the internal hernial opening to close the defect. A patch of polypropylene mesh was then placed over the internal hernial defect. After a 2-year follow-up period a recurrence rate of greater than 25% was reported [4].

A subsequent development was the transabdominal onlay patch technique. This is a relatively simple procedure which involves the intraperitoneal onlay of a prosthetic patch and securing it to the peritoneum with staples. This technique was popularized by Toy and Smoot [14] who used a patch of expanded polytetrafluoroethylene (PTFE) to cover the hernial defect. Although this technique is still used there is a concern that adhesion formation to the intra-abdominal contents and subsequent complications, for example obstruction and fistulization, may result [15].

A more recent technique is the extraperitoneal technique developed by McKernan and Laws [16] which has the advantage that the abdominal cavity is not violated. The subsequent dissection is similar to the method described in the trans-abdominal approach. The major advantage of this technique is the reduction in the incidence of complications associated with the creation of a pneumoperitoneum [17]. However, the dissection is considerably more difficult and the learning curve even longer than for the transabdominal preperitoneal approach.

Many surgeons are hesitant about using a mesh regardless of the approach, because of concern over prosthesis infection and the possibility of adhesion formation, bowel obstruction and/or fistulization. However, Lichtenstein *et al.* [18], Stoppa *et al.* [19] and Nyhus *et al.* [20] have reported extensive series of preperitoneal hernia repair using non-absorbable material with very low rates of infection. In addition, if the mesh is covered following laparoscopic insertion then the incidence of adhesion or fistula formation should be reduced.

We strongly believe that one of the most important aspects of performing a laparoscopic repair is the identification of key anatomical landmarks. Certain anatomical structures such as the iliopubic tract, Cooper's ligament, lateral border of the rectus and the transversus abdominus arch should be clearly identified. The mesh should be stapled in a curtain fashion; the most inferomedial border is stapled to Cooper's ligament, and the medial border overlaps the lateral border of the rectus to which it is stapled. The superior edge is stapled to the transversus abdominus arch. The lateral border is stapled down to the iliopubic tract. No staples should be inserted below the iliopubic tract, which is the critical landmark. Any staples below this structure could injure the external iliac vessels, or the lateral cutaneous nerve of the thigh laterally. We feel that the mesh should be at least 1–2 cm beyond the lateral border of the rectus medially and covering the angle between the inferior epigastric vessels and the lateral border of the rectus superiorly. In patients with large indirect hernia it is difficult to assess the posterior wall of the inguinal canal and the presence or absence of a coexisting direct hernia. Consequently a large piece of mesh covering the lateral border of the rectus should be used.

We have had two recurrences to date seen in the early part of the series. In patients who undergo a laparoscopic repair it is important to realize that this is a tension-free mesh repair and the defect is still present. Following dissection blood may track into the defect and give the impression of an irreducible recurrent hernia. This presented as such in one of our patients who underwent surgical exploration to rule out apparent strangulation. Ultrasound may assist in the identification of such a collection and we have found that these haematomas resolve spontaneously.

We have also noted that most of the patients who have undergone a laparoscopic hernia repair for direct hernias continue to have a cough impulse in the immediate postoperative period until sufficient fibrosis has occurred at the site of the hernia, which usually takes 4–6 weeks. We now counsel the patient preoperatively and emphasize that they will continue to have a bulge for the initial period of time.

Two patients in this series presented within 48 h following surgery with paraesthesia over the distribution of the lateral cutaneous nerve of the thigh. In both cases the symptoms resolved spontaneously within 2 weeks of the procedure following therapy with non-steroidal anti-inflammatory drugs. This has been one of the more common complications reported with laparoscopic inguinal hernia repair [21]. The most serious complication in this series was a small bowel obstruction after the herniation of a small portion of bowel between two staples. This has been a recognized complication of the TAPP repair [22]. This complication led to the only mortality in our series. We believe that violation of the peritoneum in a TAPP repair is likely to leave this approach inherently susceptible to adhesive small bowel obstruction regardless of meticulous surgical technique. This raises the question as to whether a totally extraperitoneal approach to hernia repair would be a more attractive alternative as complications such as this could be avoided.

In summary, laparoscopic inguinal hernia repair could represent an attractive alternative to conventional open inguinal hernia repair. However, it has to be shown to have less postoperative morbidity and obviously a decrease in the long-term recurrence rate. The follow-up of this series is quite short and to address the question of recurrence we feel that a multicentre prospective randomized trial is warranted. We feel that future studies are required to determine whether the benefits outweigh the disadvantages of converting an extraperitoneal hernia repair under local anaesthesia to one requiring general anaesthesia.

References

1 Nyhus LM, Bombeck CT. *Hernias*. In Sabiston DC (ed.) *Textbook of Surgery*, 13th edn. WB Saunders, Philadelphia, 1986: 1321–1352.
2 Arregui M, Davis C, Yucel O, Nagan R. Laparoscopic mesh repair of inguinal hernia using a preperitoneal approach: a preliminary report. *Surg Laparosc Endosc* 1992; **2**(1): 53–58.

3 Newman L, Eubanks S, Mason E, Duncan TD. Is laparoscopic herniorrhaphy an effective alternative to open hernia repair? *J Laparoendosc Surg* 1993; **3**: 121–128.

4 Corbitt JD. Transabdominal preperitoneal herniorrhaphy. *Surg Laparosc Endosc* 1993; **4**: 328–332.

5 Cuschieri A, Dubois F, Mouiel J *et al.* The European experience with laparoscopic cholecystectomy. *Am J Surg* 1991; **161**: 385–387.

6 Ganey JB, Johnson PA, Prillman PE, McSwain GR. Cholecystectomy: clinical experience with a large series. *Ann J Surg* 1986; **156**: 352–357.

7 McSherry CK. Cholecystectomy: the gold standard. *Am J Surg* 1989; **158**: 174–178.

8 Pickleman J, Gonzalez RP. The improving results of cholecystectomy. *Arch Surg* 1986; **121**: 930–934.

9 Rutkow IM. Surgical operations and manpower: can technical proficiency be maintained? In *Socioeconomics of Surgery*. CV Mosby, St Louis, 1989: 16–17.

10 Wantz GE. Complications of inguinal hernia repair. *Surg Clin North Am* 1984; **64**: 287–298.

11 Ger R, Monroe K, Duvivier R *et al.* Management of indirect inguinal hernias by laparoscopic closure of the neck of the sac. *Am J Surg* 1990; **159**: 370.

12 Schultz L, Graber J, Pietrafitta J *et al.* Laser laparoscopic herniorrhaphy: A clinical trial: Preliminary results. *J Laparoendosc Surg* 1990; **1**: 41.

13 Corbitt JD. Laparoscopic herniorrhaphy. *Surg Laparosc Endosc* 1991; **1**: 23.

14 Toy FK, Smoot RT Jr. Toy–Smoot laparoscopic hernioplasty. *Surg Laparosc Endosc* 1991; **1**: 151.

15 MacFadyen BV, Arregui ME, Corbitt JD, Filipi CJ, Fitzgibbons RJ *et al.* Complications of laparoscopic herniorrhaphy. *Surg Endosc* 1993; **7**: 155–158.

16 McKernan BJ, Laws HL. Laparoscopic preperitoneal prosthetic repair of inguinal hernias. *Surgical Rounds* 1992; **15**: 579–610.

17 Ponsky J. Complications of laparoscopic cholecystectomy. *Am J Surg* 1991; **161**: 393–397.

18 Lichtenstein IL, Shulman AG, Amid PK *et al.* The tension free hernioplasty. *Am J Surg* 1989; **157**: 188–192.

19 Stoppa RE, Rives JL, Warlaumont CR *et al.* The use of Dacron in the repair of hernias of the groin. *Surg Clin North Am* 1984; **64**: 269.

20 Nyhus LM, Pollack R, Bombeck CT *et al.* The preperitoneal approach and prosthetic buttress repair for recurrent hernia. *Ann Surg* 1988; **208**: 733.

21 Kraus MA. Nerve injury during laparoscopic inguinal hernia repair. *Surg Laparosc Endosc* 1993; **3**: 342–345.

22 Hendrickse CW, Evans DS. Intestinal obstruction following laparoscopic inguinal hernia repair. *Br J Surg* 1993; **80**: 1432.

Chapter 7

TAPP repair: the Hull and Stockport experience

W. Brough and C. Royston

Hernia is a very common condition affecting 3–8% of the population. Approximately 80 000 hernia repairs are performed each year in the United Kingdom [1]. Many different authors have reported different methods for repair of inguinal hernia and this possibly reflects that there are defects in these methods which give less than satisfactory results. We have to be clear on the objectives of the operations in order to assess the efficacy of the particular operation. The aim of inguinal hernia repair is to achieve a sound repair with minimal time in hospital, minimal time to full recovery and the lowest recurrence rate.

Many methods of repair have been proposed, each claiming to achieve good results. These have included darns [2], transversalis plication [3], preperitoneal mesh repair [4], and tension-free hernioplasty [5]. Early reports of laparoscopic hernia repair are now available [6, 7]. Unfortunately some surgeons have not incorporated the lessons learnt from previous research into hernia surgery. Consequently there are a plethora of techniques described, some of which are associated with a high early recurrence rate.

History

In 1884 Bassini reported an extraperitoneal groin approach to inguinal hernia repair [8] which has dominated surgical thinking for most of this century. Many modifications were suggested by Halstead, McEvedy, and McVay [8] to avoid testicular complications. Despite these modifications it is now accepted that the recurrence rate for this type of repair is unacceptably high. Recent collected series from around the world employing the Bassini repair or its modifications report recurrence rates of 0–7% for indirect, 1–10% for direct, and 5–35% for recurrent hernias. In addition to recurrence, painful postoperative neuromas, spermatic cord injury, bruising and ischaemic orchitis are occasionally seen with extraperitoneal groin herniorrhaphy [9]. Marcy emphasized the importance of high ligation of the sac in order to prevent recurrence [10]. In 1982 Ger [11] reported repair of inguinal hernias through an abdominal approach placing Michelle clips on the neck of the sac rather than performing a high ligation. More recently Corbitt has described the technique for the transperitoneal repair of inguinal hernias laparoscopically [6]. Since these early reports many different methods have been used including a mesh plug in the inguinal sac and repairs using mesh in the preperitoneal space. Some preperitoneal mesh methods may use mesh cut to fit around the cord structures whereas others use a single piece of mesh. In addition to the developments in laparoscopic techniques there have been reports of the tension-free hernioplasty from the Lichtenstein clinic using an open mesh prosthetic repair [5]. This method, employing a Prolene mesh placed in the inguinal canal tested in a large series of patients, has a very low recurrence rate and will no doubt become the 'gold standard' by which all other repairs will be assessed.

Following the successful introduction of laparoscopic cholecystectomy attentions have turned to laparoscopic inguinal hernia repair. Initial reports mainly from America described a 'plug prosthesis', usually of prolene mesh, to fill the inguinal sac and canal to induce fibrosis. Unfortunately this repair had a high incidence of early recurrence and has largely been replaced by the preperitoneal mesh repair. This might have been predicted from our previous understanding of hernia recurrence as this method makes no attempt at high ligation of the sac as advocated by Marcy.

From the conception of our series we have endeavoured to perform a preperitoneal mesh repair similar to that described by Stoppa and Nyhus [4, 9]. As with all laparoscopic procedures, the principles of the surgical procedure should not be compromised nor the lessons of previous researchers be forgotten in order to allow the operation to be carried out laparoscopically.

Our method is based on the following principles aimed at achieving a low recurrence rate.

1 *High ligation of the sac.* Marcy [10] realized that, if the sac was not ligated high, there would be an increased chance of recurrence. This is probably the explanation for the high recurrence rate seen with the 'plug mesh' repair as no attempt is made to deal with the sac.

2 *Complete dissection of the preperitoneal space.* Fruchaud realized that all hernias were a result of a defect in the musculopectineal opening irrespective of their superficial opening [12]. He postulated that the distinction between femoral and inguinal hernias was pointless since the same mechanism accounted for both defects. It is thought that the weak area of the musculopectineal opening, the transversalis fascia and its analogues, represent the only resistant layer of the abdominal wall. This is the best layer for inguinal hernia repairs in which the wall must be sutured without tension or reinforced. It was Stoppa who demonstrated that behind the transversalis fascia is a wide cleavable cellular space that communicates to a similar space on the other side via the retropubic space known as the 'cave of Retzius'. This dissection allows the vas deferens and the spermatic vessels to be mobilized from the peritoneum, termed by Stoppa as parietalization of the vessels, thereby making the vas and vessels extraperitoneal. This dissection allows accurate placing of a single piece of preperitoneal mesh that does not require cutting to allow fitting around the cord structures. In addition, as pointed out by Stoppa [13], this retrofascial space communicates with the other side allowing the simple repair of bilateral inguinal hernias with one piece of prosthetic mesh.

The method we have adopted aims at careful dissection of the sac away from the cord and is the modern equivalent of a high ligation of the sac. The dissection continues in this preperitoneal retrofascial space separating the vas and the vessels from the peritoneum, so-called parietalization, which in turn results in the cord being placed lateral to its natural position. When dissection of the preperitoneal space is complete then accurate placement of the prosthetic mesh can be achieved. This allows strengthening of the transversalis fascia and repair of the defects. By adopting this method we hope to achieve the long-term results of other series using mesh repairs but with the additional benefit of the faster rehabilitation associated with laparoscopic repair.

Method

Laparoscopic inguinal hernia repair is carried out under general anaesthetic. The patient is placed supine on the operating table and given an intravenous dose of a cephalosporin at induction because a prosthesis is to be used. The patient is encouraged to pass urine at the time of premedication to avoid the need for catheterization. The skin is prepared with antiseptic solution to prevent infection which is of importance, again because a prosthesis is being used. Insufflation is carried out in the usual way at the umbilicus with a Veress needle. After confirming that the Veress needle is in the peritoneum by aspiration and the 'saline drop test', insufflation is carried out until 4 litres of carbon dioxide have been introduced. A 10 mm cannula is introduced at the umbilicus and the camera passed into the peritoneal cavity to allow a full laparoscopic inspection of the abdominal cavity. One advantage of the transperitoneal approach to inguinal hernia repair is that both hernial orifices may be examined. In several cases we have found an undiagnosed hernia of the other side which can then be repaired at the same time. After careful examination of the abdominal contents and the hernial orifices, a 5 mm cannula is place in the same side as the hernia in the mid-clavicular line at the level of the umbilicus. On the opposite side to the hernia a 12.5 mm cannula is placed again in the mid-clavicular line at the level of the umbilicus. When the diagnosis has been confirmed, the dissection of the preperitoneal space can begin.

Indirect inguinal hernia

An indirect hernial sac is partially or fully reduced by a grasping forceps placed through the cannula on the right side of the patient. A second grasping forceps is then placed onto the superior portion of the sac and the remaining sac fully reduced using the surgeon's left hand. The grasping forceps in the surgeon's right hand is then removed and changed for a pair of diathermy scissors which are used to incise the peritoneum over the superolateral aspect of the sac. This ensures that there are no structures, in particular the inferior epigastric vessels, that can be damaged. As soon as the small incision is made into the peritoneum, carbon dioxide diffuses into the preperitoneal space aiding dissection. The peritoneum is divided over the anterior aspect of the hernial sac. We have found hydro-dissection of the preperitoneal space to be of no advantage. When this dissection is complete, the peritoneum is divided laterally, the dissection being taken towards the anterior–superior iliac spine. The resultant large incision in the peritoneum subsequently facilitates dissection of the cord contents from the sac. The thin areolar tissue of the preperitoneal space is now divided with a combination of blunt and sharp diathermy dissection. The tissues are swept back until the lateral margin of the sac is defined. The dissection now continues, pulling the anterior aspect of the sac to the patient's lateral side. This enables the dissection of the medial aspect of the sac to be performed. The peritoneum is dissected further medially, often crossing the obliterated umbilical artery. Blunt dissection again allows definition of the medial edge of the sac.

At the end of this phase the sac has been fully dissected anteriorly, medially and laterally. There is only the posterior aspect of the sac which is in close proximity to the testicular vessels and the vas deferens that requires further dissection. This is performed by grasping the anterior aspect of the sac with the grasping forceps from the 12.5 mm port and carefully stripping the structures from the posterior aspect of the sac. Thus the testicular vessels and vas deferens are teased away from the posterior aspect of the sac. This process is continued until a window develops between the sac and the cord structures. When this has been achieved, if the whole of the sac is not being removed, the peritoneum of the sac is divided and the proximal part of the sac is pulled into the abdominal cavity. Careful dissection of the testicular vessels and the vas deferens is then performed freeing the testicular vessels and the vas deferens from the peritoneum sweeping on to the posterior abdominal wall. This dissection is taken fairly high up on to the abdominal wall so that the mesh can be placed into this position. The dissection of the posterior peritoneum is continued laterally and medially. It is particularly important to free the vas deferens completely as it swings anteriorly to pass around the obliterated umbilical vein and the inferior epigastric artery. Numerous small adhesions from the peritoneum to the vas deferens must be divided to allow the mesh to settle snugly into the true preperitoneal space. When this phase is complete, the anterolateral aspect of the peritoneum is freed to separate the peritoneum from the underlying transversus muscle and to free the peritoneum around the deep ring and inferior epigastric vessels.

The final phase of the dissection is to identify the pubic ramus and pubic tubercle. This is done by placing a pair of closed forceps immediately lateral to the obliterated umbilical artery and sweeping the tissues medially, thus putting traction on the tissues over the pubic ramus. With dissecting scissors from the opposite cannula, blunt dissection enables the pubic ramus to be identified. Once the glistening fibres of the periosteum over the pubic ramus are identified, the ramus can be traced up to the pubic tubercle which is in turn exposed. Care must be taken whilst performing this manoeuvre in case an abnormal obturator artery is present which will be seen running down from the inferior epigastric vessels to enter the obturator foramen after passing over the femoral canal. When the dissection is complete, a piece of Prolene mesh measuring 15×10 cm is rolled up like a cigarette and, after 'back loading' the mesh into the reducing sleeve with the grasping forceps, introduced into the 12.5 mm cannula. It is not necessary to draw a longitudinal line on the mesh for orientation purposes. The mesh is positioned so that it lies longitudinally across the inguinal region. It is imperative to place the mesh so that it completely covers the area of Hasselbach's triangle and the deep inguinal ring. The mesh is then stapled, firstly to the pubic tubercle and a further three staples into the inferior pubic ramus;

a further staple is placed immediately medial to the inferior epigastric artery, the next staple lateral to the inferior epigastric artery. This ensures that the mesh covers the whole of Hasselbach's triangle and the deep inguinal ring. A further staple is inserted to fix the lateral aspect of the mesh superiorly. It is important not to place staples into the psoas muscle laterally as this may trap the lateral cutaneous nerve of the thigh resulting in a meralgia paraesthetica.

When the mesh is stapled into the correct position, the peritoneum is lifted up over the mesh so that the mesh lies snugly over the testicular vessels and the vas deferens. The peritoneum is then closed with a series of staples. There are often small gaps between the staples but these will close as the peritoneum is allowed to collapse. It is our practice to instill bupivacaine 1 mg/kg into the preperitoneal space. When the closure of the peritoneum is completed, the cannulae are removed. The 10 and 12.5 mm cannulae sites are closed with Vicryl under direct vision and 4/0 subcuticular pds to skin. The 5 mm cannula site is closed with steristrips.

Female inguinal hernia

In the case of female inguinal hernias a basic anatomical difference affects the dissection while allowing the same repair to be performed. This is the round ligament, which needs to be parietalized instead of the vas and spermatic vessels. The round ligament extends from the junction of the uterus and fallopian tube to the deep inguinal ring. It lies in the anterior leaf of the broad ligament and is covered by peritoneum on all sides. The round ligament passes through the deep inguinal ring to reach the inguinal canal and is attached at its distal extremity to the fibro-fatty tissue of the labium majus of the vulva. It is supplied by the ovarian artery and a branch of the inferior epigastric artery in the inguinal canal. In order to carry out a dissection of the preperitoneal space it is necessary to dissect out the round ligament fully with the sac until it enters the inguinal canal. It is important to trace the ligament to its origin at the junction of the uterus and the fallopian tube where it can be transected with diathermy scissors to leave no structures traversing the preperitoneal space. A 15×10 cm Prolene mesh can then be stapled into the preperitoneal space as previously described.

Direct inguinal hernia

Cannula position for a direct inguinal hernia is identical to that for an indirect inguinal hernia. Dissection commences at the superior aspect of the direct hernia. After reduction of the sac by grasping forceps, the peritoneum is divided along the extent of the sac, then laterally, over the obliterated umbilical artery, continuing through the deep inguinal ring and out towards the anterior–superior iliac spine. The peritoneum is next reflected off the testicular vessels and vas deferens. This is easier than with an indirect inguinal hernia as there is no indirect sac to dissect free from the cord structures. When this has been accomplished, the peritoneum of the direct hernia is completely dissected free. At this stage it is important to appreciate that there is a clear tissue plane between the peritoneum forming the direct hernial sac and the transversalis fascia. This plane must be entered to allow the transversalis fascia to free and prolapse anteriorly while the true peritoneum of the sac is withdrawn into the abdomen. Unless this dissection is carried out correctly it will not be possible to define the margins of the direct hernia and therefore allow accurate placement of the mesh. The peritoneum and any fatty tissue is completely removed from the hernial defect. Prolene mesh measuring 15×10 cm is inserted into the inguinal region as described for indirect inguinal hernia and stapled in the same way. It is very important to make sure that the mesh completely covers the area of the direct hernia. The mesh must be lifted well anteriorly towards the arcuate line of Douglas to make sure that the covering is complete. The peritoneum is closed as before.

Sliding hernia

With a sliding hernia the sigmoid colon or caecum is in very close proximity to the peritoneum at the level of the deep inguinal ring. Care must be taken to ensure that the bowel is not damaged whilst mobilizing the peritoneum at this level. The dissection is very similar to that of an indirect inguinal hernia. As soon as an incision is made into the peritoneum carbon dioxide diffuses into the area and the peritoneal dissection is extended laterally towards the anterior–superior iliac spine. When this has been performed it is extended medially and the peritoneum is reflected off the testicular vessels and the vas deferens, the sigmoid colon or caecum being mobilized at the same time. The same landmarks as for an indirect inguinal hernia are identified and the Prolene mesh measuring 15×10 cm is inserted into the preperitoneal space and stapled as previously described. Care must be taken when closing the peritoneum over the mesh as the sigmoid colon or caecum will be brought up with the thin edge of peritoneum in order to obtain closure, and it is clearly imperative to ensure that no staples are put into the bowel whilst closing the peritoneum.

With each of the above closures, if a very large defect is present, it may be necessary to use a larger piece of Prolene mesh to ensure that the area is completely covered. We have not attempted to mould the mesh in any way and we have always laid the mesh on to the peritoneal aspect of the testicular vessels and the vas deferens; however, it is very important to ensure that the peritoneal dissection is carried out well posteriorly exposing the iliac vessels to enable the mesh to be inserted without the lower border of the mesh rolling up.

Recurrent inguinal hernia

Recurrent inguinal hernias are particularly suitable for laparoscopic repair. The principal advantage of repairing recurrent inguinal hernias laparoscopically is that dissection occurs in virgin territory. A recurrent hernia usually has a very well-defined fibrous margin which can be easily covered with a Prolene mesh. The peritoneum of the recurrent hernia is grasped and reduced into the abdominal cavity. The peritoneum is incised on the superior margin of the recurrent sac with diathermy scissors. The peritoneum is dissected along the length of the recurrent hernia and then across the obliterated umbilical artery, the deep inguinal ring and towards the pubic tubercle. The dissection is therefore identical to that of indirect and direct inguinal hernias. When the peritoneum has been dissected free from the testicular vessels and the vas deferens, and the pubic tubercle and the pubic ramus have been identified, Prolene mesh again measuring 15×10 cm is inserted to the inguinal preperitoneal space and fixed using staples to the previously described structures. Occasionally, it may be necessary to place some additional staples around the fibrous ring of the recurrent defect. The peritoneum is then closed.

Femoral hernia

It is not our policy to consider femoral hernias suitable for laparoscopic mesh repair as in the elective situation a Lothesin 'low approach' is a minor procedure with a rapid recovery and low morbidity. However, should a femoral hernia be recognized at laparoscopy with or without an associated inguinal hernia then the standard dissection with mesh repair as described above will cover the femoral canal after reduction of the hernial contents. It should be remembered that the dissection is taking place adjacent to the external iliac vein as the immediate lateral relation and is at risk of damage during dissection and reduction of the sac contents.

Obturator hernia

This type of hernia will occasionally be diagnosed in addition to an inguinal hernia. Recognition of this type of hernia is important as the contents entering the obturator foramen must be reduced to allow the mesh to be placed in the true preperitoneal space after parietalizing the vas and vessels.

Bilateral inguinal hernia repair (Bikini mesh repair)

Bilateral inguinal hernias are ideally suited for laparoscopic mesh repair. The great advantage of the laparoscopic approach is that it avoids the scrotal and penile oedema which is so common after bilateral open repairs. The pain from a bilateral laparoscopic inguinal hernia repair is the same as that of a single hernia repair, the main discomfort coming from the cannula sites rather than the inguinal region itself.

The patient is placed on the operating table in the supine position. Catheterization of the bladder is not necessary as all patients are asked to void urine at the time of premedication. Insufflation is performed as for a single hernia repair via the umbilicus, and a 10 mm cannula with telescope is inserted. The presence of bilateral inguinal hernias is confirmed and two 12.5 mm cannulae are inserted at the midclavicular line at the level of the umbilicus. Dissection of both hernial sacs and inguinal regions are performed as previously described. When both preperitoneal spaces of the inguinal regions have been dissected so that the peritoneum has been stripped off the testicular vessels and vas deferens, a long curved forceps is inserted in the right-hand 12.5 mm cannula and passed immediately behind the pubic symphysis to the preperitoneal space of the opposite side. The tips of the forceps are thus seen near the left pubic tubercle. The 'cave of Retzius' is then opened up and the loose areolar tissue behind the rectus muscle is dissected free, opening up a large space. A piece of Prolene mesh measuring 28 × 10 cm is rolled up like a cigarette and inserted into the left-hand 12.5 mm cannula. One end of this mesh is then fed into the open forceps that have been placed across the 'cave of Retzius' and the mesh is pulled through from the left to the right preperitoneal space. The mesh therefore lies in the immediate suprapubic region passing behind the pubic symphysis. The mesh is positioned so that equal lengths are present on each side and it is opened out and stapled to cover Hasselbach's triangle and the deep inguinal ring on each side. Staples are then inserted into the pubic ramus, pubic tubercle, and each side of each inferior epigastric vessel. The peritoneum is then closed as for unilateral repairs. This procedure, depending on the patient's age, can be satisfactorily performed as a day-case procedure. All of the cannula sites are closed with Vicryl under direct vision and 4/0 subcuticular pds to skin.

Laparoscopic repair of laparoscopic recurrent hernia

To date there have been patients with recurrent hernia developing after laparoscopic repair at nearly 2 years (recurrence rate approximately 1%). In four of these cases, the patients elected to have a further laparoscopic mesh repair of the recurrent hernia. One patient had an open repair as the hernia disappeared after micturition. Open surgery confirmed a recurrence containing bladder.

In each of the four patients that underwent laparoscopic repair a small medial recurrence was noted. The mesh had rolled up from the inferior ramus leaving the medial end of the inguinal canal exposed. In all cases a mature peritoneal sac had reformed and in some cases actually contained bowel. It is interesting to note that at this second laparoscopy the mesh had been completely reperitonealized.

The method we use to repair a recurrence following laparoscopic herniorrhaphy is to reduce the sac and re-enter the preperitoneal space medially over the ramus and the symphysis pubis. The dissection is continued until the sac has been separated from the transversalis fascia. At this stage we usually find the rolled-up mesh in the region of the inferior epigastric vessels. This rolled-up mesh plug needs to be excised as it is often contained within the hernia preventing a satisfactory repair. The medial edge of the original mesh is then exposed, precluding the need for dissection further lateral. A second piece of mesh is then introduced in the normal way and placed with the medial edge past the midline of the symphysis pubis, making sure that the mesh is pulled up towards the arcuate line of Douglas. The second piece of mesh is then stapled into place with an overlap with the medial edge of the first piece of mesh. Staples are placed into the 'double-breasted' piece of mesh. There is usually sufficient peritoneum from the sac to allow the mesh to be completely reperitonealized. Recovery is similar to that for normal laparoscopic hernia repair and we await the long-term results.

The lessons learnt from carrying out laparoscopy on patients with recurrent hernia are as follows:

1 We have increased the size of the mesh from the initial 11 × 6 cm to 15 × 10 cm or larger if necessary. This is in the belief that with a greater surface area of mesh there is less pressure tending to displace the mesh. In addition, with experience the area of dissection has increased as our understanding of the anatomy has also increased.

2 We now place three staples into the inferior pubic ramus as it would appear that part of the mechanism for recurrence is the mesh rolling up from the ramus. Initially we used one staple and we feel that this is insufficient.

3 We feel that in common with the Lichtenstein mesh repair the mesh should be placed medially to the symphysis and not just to the pubic tubercle.

Postoperative care

Patients may eat and drink as soon as they are recovered from the anaesthetic. Patients are usually discharged the same day or after an overnight stay depending on the patient. There are few objections on clinical grounds to discharging a patient on the same day as surgery. No specific instructions are given other than that they may continue normal activities as soon as they feel comfortable. There is a lot of sense in the adage 'if it hurts don't do it'.

Results

We have carried out laparoscopic hernia repairs in 500 patients using the transperitoneal preperitoneal mesh repair. There were 489 males and 11 female patients with a median age of 54 years (range 17–83 years). The breakdown of the classification of the hernia repairs is given in Table 7.1. None of the operations was performed for irreducible or obstructed inguinal hernias.

Postoperative course

Most patients were discharged after an overnight stay with no complications and returned to normal activity in a very short time. A total of 66 patients underwent

Table 7.1

Spread of patients undergoing transperitoneal preperitoneal mesh repairs.

	No. of patients	% of patients
Indirect inguinal hernia	382	76
Direct inguinal hernia	183	36
Pantaloon hernia	27	5.4
Recurrent inguinal hernia		
Indirect	11	2.2
Direct	38	7.6
Bilateral inguinal hernia	82	16
Sliding hernia	23	4.6

laparoscopic hernia repair as a day case (13%) while 393 remained in hospital as a planned overnight stay (89%). 37 patients required a two-night hospital stay (8.4%) and 11 patients went home after three nights or more (2.5%).

A total of 122 patients had a previous hernia repair, while 43 patients had appendicectomy. Laparotomy had been performed in 27 patients and 13 patients had a previous vasectomy. These histories of previous surgery did not affect our ability to carry out laparoscopic inguinal hernia repair.

For the group undergoing unilateral repair, including recurrent hernia repair, the median time to return to normal activity was 5 days (range 1–42 days). This was measured by the time to driving a car in most cases or where not applicable patients were questioned as to their return to normal activity. These variables have been used in other hernia series. In contrast, the return to normal activity for the 82 patients after bilateral inguinal hernia repair was a median of 7 days (range 2–28 days).

The return to work for the two groups was assessed only in those patients who were not retired or unemployed. For the unilateral group the median return to work was 13 days (range 2–90 days) and for the bilateral group 14 days (range 2–56 days). Overall these results would suggest that it is possible to obtain a rapid recovery following laparoscopic inguinal hernia repair. In addition, the bilateral group recover in a similar time to the unilateral group.

Complications

Laparoscopy and insufflation

There were no complications from insufflation in this series. This is an important fact as one of the major criticisms of this technique is that if there is a problem then a laparotomy may be required to deal with the complication. This would not be acceptable in modern hernia surgery as good results can be obtained from other techniques.

Intestinal obstruction

There were two cases of bowel obstruction in this series. The underlying cause in each case was different. The first was due to incisional herniation of a lateral port site. Herniation at laparoscopy is rare. Although the true incidence is unknown, it has been estimated at 0.07% and the criticism made by advocates of open hernia repair would be that this complication would never happen with a traditional repair. We take care to close all port sites of 10 mm and greater.

In the second case the patient underwent immediate laparoscopy using the Hasson technique. We found that the peritoneal closure over the mesh had become separated and a knuckle of small bowel was trapped beneath a flap of peritoneum. This may have resulted from distension from the patient having acute retention of urine postoperatively. The bowel was reduced laparoscopically and the peritoneum closed with an uneventful recovery. This confirms our belief in accurate closure of the peritoneum after placement of the mesh.

Haemorrhage

We have not encountered any major haemorrhage in this series. In two cases we have seen bleeding as a result of damage to the inferior epigastric vessels but this was easily controlled with clips and was of no consequence. Fortunately we have not had any damage to the external iliac vessels but to avoid this complication we always start our peritoneal incision superolateral thus avoiding any major structures until the true preperitoneal space is entered.

Bruising

There tends to be less bruising after laparoscopic hernia repair than in traditional repair. In this series we had six patients who reported bruising following surgery. However, in the follow-up clinic at 1 week no patients examined had visible bruising, suggesting that the patients' reports were of minor discoloration.

Damage to cord structures

Unilateral vasectomy occurred in two cases. In one of these cases there appeared to be damage to the testicular artery. The patient was in pain for a few days but then settled. To the present date there do not appear to be signs of testicular atrophy. It has been suggested that if the artery to the vas deferens is intact then sufficient blood supply remains. A total of 17 patients reported testicular pain of varying severity and duration. However, in all cases this has been self-limiting by the first follow-up appointment between 4 and 6 weeks postoperatively.

Damage to viscera

We have not experienced to date any damage to viscera or vessels as a result of laparoscopy or dissection of the preperitoneal space. We acknowledge that this is always a potential hazard and we always take care to insufflate with 4 litres of carbon dioxide prior to placing the first cannula.

Urinary retention

Only five patients suffered acute retention of urine following laparoscopic hernia repair. This we found to be surprisingly low. Two patients went on to require transurethal prostatectomy. We would have predicted on past experience of hernia repairs in this elderly population and the large number of bilateral hernia repairs that this complication would have been more common.

Swollen testicles

Only one patient reported a swollen testicle, which settled by the postoperative follow-up appointment. We can only postulate that damage to the vascular supply to the testis may have occurred but to date the patient has made a full recovery with no evidence of testicular atrophy.

Seromas

There were no postoperative hydroceles detected but a total of 49 seromas were identified and treated by simple aspiration. The seroma presents with a lump in the groin and is often mistaken for an early recurrence of the hernia. In fact the lump feels like 'a hard boiled egg' and on examination it is possible to get above the lump. Simple aspiration usually reassures both the surgeon and patient with full resolution of the cystic collection.

Wound infection

Six patients reported port site redness but no overt wound infections were noted requiring drainage or readmission to hospital. All port sites are sutured and to date there have been no port site hernias reported.

Meralgia paraesthetica

Eleven patients have developed meralgia paraesthetica over the distribution of the lateral cutaneous nerve of the thigh. In all cases this has been self-limiting within 6 weeks of surgery with the patients returning to full activity. We have learnt to avoid this complication by not placing the staple too far laterally and inferior near the psoas muscle. We have not observed any other nerve damage. Thus far no patients have required removal of the mesh for this condition although occasionally the symptoms can be distressing and require strong analgesia for a considerable time. From our limited experience of repairing recurrent hernias after laparoscopic mesh repair, we would not recommend mesh removal as this would be technically very difficult since the mesh is adherent to surrounding structures. In addition we feel that damage to the major vessels may occur very easily while attempting to remove the mesh.

Recurrence

A total of five patients have confirmed recurrent hernias and these have been repaired; follow-up of these patients will give us insight into the possible mechanism of recurrence. Only one patient elected to have the recurrent hernia repaired traditionally and the remaining four patients have undergone a further laparoscopic repair.

Mesh infection

It is our practice to give all patients one dose of intravenous antibiotics at the time of insufflation as a prosthesis is being introduced. We have one patient who presented 6 months after surgery with a small abscess in the groin. An incision was made over the abscess; the sterile pus was drained and in addition the prosthetic mesh 'floated' out of the abscess cavity. There was no sign of recurrent hernia. The wound healed satisfactorily.

Discussion

We have adopted the laparoscopic mesh repair for inguinal hernia in 500 patients. In all cases we have removed all or most of the sac in order to reduce the hernia. It was established by Marcy that if the sac was not ligated high there would be an increased recurrence rate. In our method we have carried out a tension-free repair in order to achieve results comparable to other large series of mesh repair when placed at conventional surgery. This relatively pain-free procedure allows rapid rehabilitation. There are, nevertheless, many issues for debate which are not in the remit of this chapter. However, it would not be right if we could not defend our reasoning for choosing this particular method of repair.

Many authors have shown that traditional tension repair of the Bassini type is associated with a high recurrence rate of approximately 15–20%. Many surgeons do not accept this fact but, unfortunately, owing to poor self-audit, cannot refute these figures. The tension-free mesh repair is associated with a low recurrence rate (2%). With laparoscopic placement of the mesh we hope to achieve early rehabilitation and a low recurrence rate. In our series it is too early to look seriously at the recurrence rate but the early results are encouraging. We have five recurrences to date after 2 years from 500 cases but expect this figure to increase for two reasons. Firstly, these initial results include the learning curve of the surgeons concerned and over the past 2 years our technique has been modified whereby we make a larger dissection of the preperitoneal space and use a larger piece of mesh. We are confident the method is scientifically sound and the same as open tension-free mesh repair. The distinct advantages that we have found to both the surgeon and the patient is in the case of the recurrent and bilateral inguinal hernia. In the former the operation is being carried out in virgin tissue planes and is very easy to perform. The tension-free mesh repair allows a very rapid recovery and the patients appear to be very pleased with the surgery when asked for a comparison with the traditional repair. In the case of the bilateral hernia repair there is a recovery time of a single hernia repair. From the surgery the operation time is very short (median time 45 min) and the single mesh passed behind the symphysis to cover both inguinal regions can easily be performed by a single surgeon. The patients are all discharged at 24 hours and return to normal activity very quickly.

The learning curve for laparoscopic tension-free mesh repair is short and the operating time is soon reduced to approximately 30 min per case. The cost of the procedures has been a major barrier to many surgeons performing this procedure on a routine basis. With the short stay, particularly for the recurrent hernia patients and the patients with bilateral hernia, the bed saving will more than justify this procedure. In addition, our results would suggest that bilateral laparoscopic inguinal hernia repair is associated with less bruising and penile oedema and a low incidence of acute retention of urine.

We have also demonstrated that the repair is associated with zero mortality and very low morbidity. Some criticisms may be levelled at us because inguinal hernia repair has now been elevated to a consultant operation. In fact this is not true and this procedure is regularly carried out by correctly trained and supervised registrars.

In conclusion, we believe that we have used evidence from previous research to formulate a logical method for the laparoscopic placement of a prosthetic mesh into the preperitoneal space. The result is a tension-free hernia repair with a rapid return to full activity. This procedure may be readily performed as a day-case procedure but does require a general anaesthetic. From our experience of teaching this procedure to many surgeons of all grades we feel that laparoscopic transperitoneal mesh repair for inguinal hernias is teachable, reproducible with a steep learning curve. With long-term follow-up of our patients we hope that the true recurrence rate associated with this procedure will be known so that surgeons will be able to make a well-balanced decision as to the type of hernia repair that they wish to offer their patients.

References

1 Kingsnorth A, Gray M, Nott D. Prospective randomised trial comparing the Shouldice technique and plication darn for inguinal hernia. *Br J Surg* 1992; **79**: 1068–1070.
2 Lifshultz H, Juler GL. The inguinal darn. *Arch Surg* 1986; **121**: 171–179.
3 Glassow F. Short stay surgery (Shouldice technique) for repair of inguinal hernia. *Ann R Coll Surg Engl* 1976; **58**: 133–139.
4 Stoppa R, Rives J, Warlaumont C, Palot J, Verhaeghe P, Delattre J. The use of Dacron in the repair of hernias of the groin. *Surg Clin North Am* 1984; **64**: 269–285.
5 Lichtenstein I, Shulman A, Amid P. The tension free hernioplasty. *Am J Surg* 1989; **157**: 188–193.
6 Corbitt JD. Laparoscopic herniorrhaphy. *Surg Laparosc Endosc* 1991; **1**: 23–25.
7 Milkins RC, Lansdown MJR, Wedgwood KR, Brough WA, Royston CMS. Laparoscopic hernia repair: a prospective study of 409 cases. *Min Invas Ther* 1993; **2**: 237–242.
8 Reed RC. Historical survey of the treatment of hernias. In Nyhus LM, Condon RE (eds) *Hernia*. JB Lippincott, Philadelphia, 1989: 1–17.
9 Condon RE, Nyhus LM. Complications of groin hernias. In Nyhus LM, Condon RE (eds) *Hernia*. JB Lippincott, Philadelphia, 1989: 253–269.
10 Marcy HO. A new use of carbolized catgut ligatures. *Boston Med Surg J* 1871; **85**: 315–316.
11 Ger R, Monroe K, Duvivier R, Mishrick A. Management of indirect inguinal hernias by laparoscopic closure of the neck of the sac. *Am J Surg* 1990; **159**: 371–373.
12 Fruchaud H. *Anatomie Chirurgicale des Hernies de l'Aine*. Doin, Paris, 1956.
13 Stoppa RE, Warlaumont CR. The preperitoneal approach and prosthetic repair of groin hernia. In Nyhus LM, Condon RE (eds) *Hernia*. JB Lippincott, Philadelphia, 1989: 199–225.

Chapter 8
Step by step TAPP repair

P.A. Paraskeva, A. Darzi and J.R.T. Monson

Many authors have described their initial experiences with this technique in small groups of patients [1–3]. In this chapter a surgical technique is described which might assist the surgeon in the laparoscopic TAPP repair and promote easier, safer and more effective laparoscopic inguinal hernia repair.

Surgical technique

Placement of the ports

All published accounts of the TAPP repair to date suggest the use of a three-port laparoscopic approach: an infraumbilical port, for the placement of the laparoscope, with two lateral ports at the level of the umbilicus for the placement of laparoscopic instruments [4]. Despite the wide acceptance of this method, our experience has found this to have three great disadvantages. Firstly, because the laparoscope is in the umbilical port and the laparoscopic tools are approaching the inguinal region from either side, the instruments tend to cross over each other and interfere with the procedure, so called 'intra-abdominal sword fighting'. Secondly, the laparoscope positioned in the umbilical port will result in the hand of the assistant always lying between those of the surgeon, therefore interfering with the surgeon during the procedure and causing an uncomfortable operating position. Finally, as many surgeons switch tools to different port sites during the procedure, the patient may be subjected to three 12 mm ports so as to accommodate any of the laparoscopic tools used in this operation, leading to three large trocar scars.

These problems can all be eradicated by implementing some simple modifications to the procedure. We also advocate a three-port laparoscopic approach when carrying out a TAPP repair. A simple and consistent arrangement of ports and port sizes is used. A 12 mm port is placed infraumbilically; a second, 10 mm, port is placed on the right side, at the level of the umbilicus. The third port, which is a 5 mm port, is placed in the left iliac fossa; its exact position in this region will vary when performing left, right or bilateral hernia repairs (Fig. 8.1). The rationale behind moving the 5 mm port is to keep the operating tools placed through the left and umbilical ports running parallel to each other when performing a right or left inguinal hernia repair. Manipulation of the tools in this fashion allows easier operating. When repairing a bilateral inguinal hernia the 5 mm port is placed between the site used for right and left inguinal hernia repair as a compromise. Therefore, whether the procedure is a left, right or bilateral hernia repair the same arrangement of ports is used. This method subjects the patient to the smallest size trocars possible, and decreases confusion in the operating room during the procedure.

Figure 8.1

Diagram of positions and sizes of ports used in a transabdominal preperitoneal patch (TAPP) repair, when repairing a left (L), right (R) and bilateral (B) inguinal hernia.

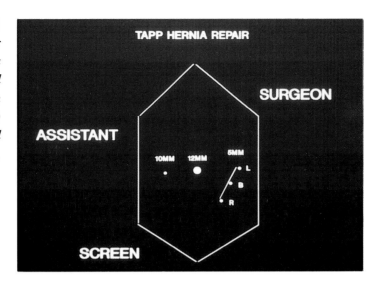

Placement of the laparoscopic instruments

The surgeon stands on the left of the patient when performing either a left, right or bilateral inguinal hernia repair. The laparoscope is always placed in the 10 mm right iliac fossa port, and is never moved from this site. The positioning of the laparoscope at this site allows good views of both the left and right inguinal regions. The 12 mm infraumbilical port is the largest port and is used for the placement of the endoscopic hernia stapler. Endoscopic scissors and graspers are also placed through this port by reducing it to a 5 mm size. The 5 mm left iliac fossa port is used for the placement of an endoscopic grasper only. The placement of the instruments in this fashion eradicates the problems associated with intra-abdominal sword fighting, as the instruments run parallel to each other and do not cross. This arrangement may also be used for repairing any type of inguinal hernia.

How to handle the prosthetic mesh

One of the most crucial aspects of repairing a hernia laparoscopically using the TAPP method is the correct positioning of the prosthetic mesh and stapling it to the underlying anatomical landmarks. This part of the procedure can be time consuming and frustrating to the surgeon. Initially, many reports advocated rolling up the mesh before placing it through the port but 'why roll if you are going to unroll?'. We propose that a corner of the prosthetic mesh should be grasped with the endoscopic grasper and then simply pushed through the infraumbilical port. The mesh is then spread out in the inguinal region and positioned over the correct anatomical landmarks. To aid in the correct positioning of the prosthetic mesh we propose the use of two endoscopic graspers: the initial one that holds the mesh through the infraumbilical port and the second through the left iliac fossa port. When repairing a right inguinal hernia, for example, the umbilical endoscopic grasper positions the initial corner of the mesh in the superolateral area of the inguinal region (Fig. 8.2). The left iliac fossa endoscopic grasper is then placed 1–2 cm medial to the umbilical grasper on the mesh (Fig. 8.3).

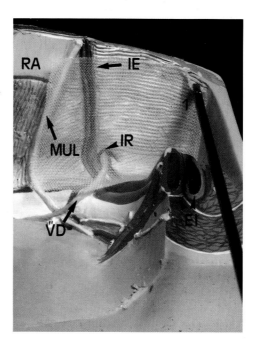

Figure 8.2

Photograph of a model of the intra-abdominal view of the right inguinal region showing the initial placement of the prosthetic mesh. RA, rectus abdominus; MUL, medial umbilical ligament; IE, inferior epigastric vessels; VD, vas deferens; IR, internal inguinal ring; EI, external iliac vessels.

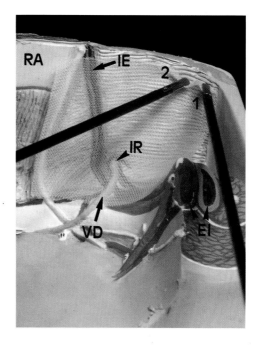

Figure 8.3

Photograph of a model of the intra-abdominal view of the right inguinal region, showing the positioning of the mesh using two endoscopic graspers. 1, first grasper; 2, second grasper; RA, rectus abdominus; IE, inferior epigastric vessels; IR, internal inguinal ring; VD, vas deferens; EI, external iliac vessels.

The initial grasper is then removed and replaced with the endoscopic hernia stapler; the initial corner is then stapled. Using the left iliac fossa grasper to hold the mesh steady, the superior border of the mesh is stapled (Fig. 8.4) followed by the medial and lateral borders (Figs 8.5–8.7). When repairing a left inguinal hernia the same principles are used except the initial corner is the superomedial corner. The use of this method of repairing inguinal hernias laparoscopically allows easier operating and accurate positioning of the mesh.

Figure 8.4

Photograph of a model of the right inguinal region showing the placement of the initial staple. RA, rectus abdominus; MUL, medial umbilical ligament; IE, inferior epigastric vessels; 2, second grasper; HS, hernia stapler; EI, external iliac vessels.

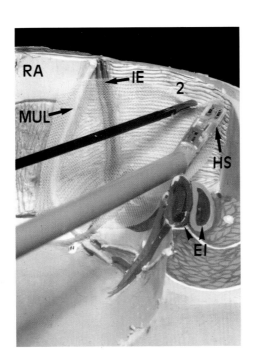

Figure 8.5

Photograph of a model of the right inguinal region showing the technique of placing the second staple along the superior edge of the prosthetic mesh. RA, rectus abdominus; IE, inferior epigastric vessels; 1, first staple; 2, second staple; HS, hernia stapler; VD, vas deferens; EI, external iliac vessels.

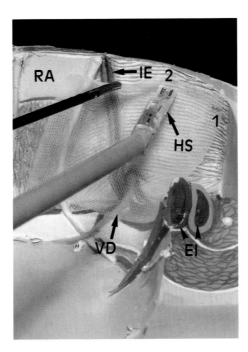

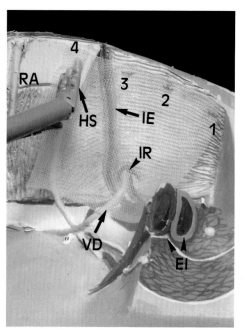

Figure 8.7
Photograph of a model of the right inguinal region showing the stapled mesh and the final staple being placed in Cooper's ligament. 1, first staple; 2, second staple; 3, third staple; 4, fourth staple; RA, rectus abdominus; HS, hernia stapler; IE, inferior epigastric vessels; IR, internal inguinal ring; VD, vas deferens; EI, external iliac vessels.

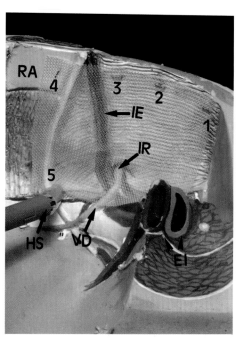

Figure 8.6
Photograph of a model of the right inguinal region showing the initial four staples in the superior edge of the prosthetic mesh. 1, first staple; 2, second staple; 3, third staple; 4 fourth staple; 5, fifth staple; RA, rectus abdominus; IE, inferior epigastric vessels; IR, internal inguinal ring; HS, hernia stapler; VD, vas deferens; EI, external iliac vessels.

Where to position the prosthetic mesh

The correct positioning of the prosthetic mesh is of vital importance if the hernia is to be repaired effectively and postoperative recurrence to be avoided. Four key anatomical landmarks should be identified: the arching fibres of transversus abdominus, the lateral border of the rectus abdominus, the iliopubic tract and Cooper's ligament. The medial border of the prosthetic mesh is stapled to the lateral border of the rectus abdominus, and the superior edge is stapled to the arching fibres of transversus abdominus. The lateral border of the mesh is stapled down to the iliopubic tract, and no further. The inferomedial corner of the mesh is stapled to Cooper's ligament. Using this technique, no staples are placed below the iliopubic tract, thereby limiting the chance of damage to structures that occur in this area. The positioning of the mesh in this fashion adequately covers the direct hernia site (Hesselbach's triangle), the indirect hernia site and the femoral hernia site, thereby decreasing the chance of postoperative recurrence. The placement of no staples below the iliopubic tract limits the chance of damage to important nerves that lie in this area, such as the lateral cutaneous nerve of the thigh [5], thereby limiting the chance of postoperative neuralgias.

Discussion

The method described for the TAPP repair of a hernia offers many advantages to both the surgeon and the patient. The use of the same trocar sites, sizes and positions regardless of the type of hernia leads to less confusion in the operating theatre. The positioning of the laparoscope in the right iliac fossa gives good views of both the right and left inguinal regions. Also, it leads to a more comfortable operating position for the surgeon and the assistant together with a clearer operating field for the surgeon. For the patient this method offers the use of the smallest trocar sizes and therefore the smallest scars.

With three-dimensional imaging emerging as a potential aid to laparoscopy, techniques that involve less crossing of instruments give a clearer picture.

This method of laparoscopic inguinal hernia repair simplifies this procedure by removing some frustrating problems, as well as offering a successful method of repair. Together with these advantages it offers the potential for conventionalizing the procedure which has important implications in the training of surgeons in laparoscopic procedures.

References

1 Arregui ME, Davis CJ, Yucel O *et al.* Laparoscopic mesh repair of inguinal hernia using a preperitoneal approach: A preliminary report. *Surg Laparosc Endosc* 1992; **2**: 53.
2 Seid AS, Deutsch H, Jacobson A. Laparoscopic herniorrhaphy. *Surg Laparosc Endosc* 1992; **2**: 59.
3 Nolen M, Melichar R, Jennings WC *et al.* Use of a Marlex fan in the repair of direct and indirect inguinal hernias by laparoscopy. *J Laparoendosc Surg* 1992; **2**: 61.
4 Corbitt JD. Transabdominal preperitoneal herniorrhaphy. *Surg Laparosc Endosc* 1993; **3**: 328–332.
5 Kraus MA. Nerve injury during laparoscopic inguinal hernia repair. *Surg Laparosc Endosc* 1993; **3**: 342–345.

Chapter 9

Extraperitoneal repair: technique and review of the literature

P.A. Paraskeva

Many surgeons believe that the future of laparoscopic hernia repair lies in the development of a totally extraperitoneal technique. The laparoscopic extraperitoneal hernia repair was first described by McKernan and Laws [1]. The term laparoscopic extraperitoneal repair is in itself a contradiction in terms, because the abdominal cavity is not entered; it is not a true laparoscopic repair. Instead the trocars and endoscopic instruments are placed in the extraperitoneal space outside the peritoneal cavity. The laparoscopic extraperitoneal repair has been proposed to be safer than other laparoscopic procedures because the complications of entering the peritoneal cavity and establishing a pneumoperitoneum are avoided [2]. It also eliminates the need to dissect intra-abdominal adhesions or manipulate the bowel. This greatly reduces the risk of bowel injury, and in addition eliminates the possibilities of adhesions of bowel to the prosthetic mesh material.

Despite these potential benefits the extraperitoneal hernia repair has not enjoyed widespread popularity. Firstly, the operating space provided is limited and requires experience with other laparoscopic procedures before it is attempted. Secondly, experience is required to become familiar with inguinal anatomy as viewed through the laparoscope from this perspective. Finally, the fixation of stapled polypropylene mesh is more difficult than with the more popular transabdominal preperitoneal technique.

Technique

The laparoscopic extraperitoneal repair is performed under general anesthesia and the patient is prepared as for a transabdominal preperitoneal hernia repair [3]. A three-trocar approach is used (Fig. 9.1): a 12 mm port is placed subumbilically, a 5 mm port is placed suprapubically in the midline, and a 10 mm port is placed in the midline between the other two. An initial incision is made subumbilically, and blunt dissection is carried out through the subcutaneous tissues down to the fascia. The rectus musculature is separated bluntly and retracted laterally. A small tunnel is then opened into the extraperitoneal space in the direction of the pubic bone between the rectus muscle. The 12 mm trocar is then placed into the extraperitoneal space (Figs 9.2–9.5). The extraperitoneal space is insufflated with carbon dioxide at a lower pressure of 12 mmHg to prevent the occurrence of acidosis or subcutaneous emphysema. The peritoneum is carefully dissected free from the anterior abdominal wall using blunt dissection under direct visualization, down to the pubic bone.

Figure 9.1

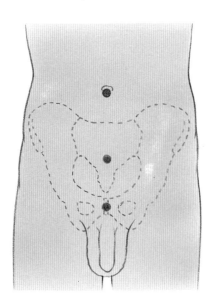

Alternatively this space could be created with the use of an extra preperitoneal balloon (Figs 9.6 and 9.9–Auto Suture, UK). Some surgeons advocate the use of an operating laparoscope to assist in the initial dissection by passing a dissecting forceps under direct vision. This dissection develops a preperitoneal tunnel for further trocar placement. Under direct vision a 10 mm trocar is placed midway between the umbilicus and the pubis, a 5 mm port is then placed suprapubically; both are placed in the midline. Formal dissection commences at the pubic symphysis and moves to the sides of the hernia along the line of Cooper's ligament. Using the additional ports the peritoneum is dissected in this direction to reveal Cooper's ligament and

Figure 9.2 (Left)
Place device.

Figure 9.3 (Right)
Remove dissector cover.

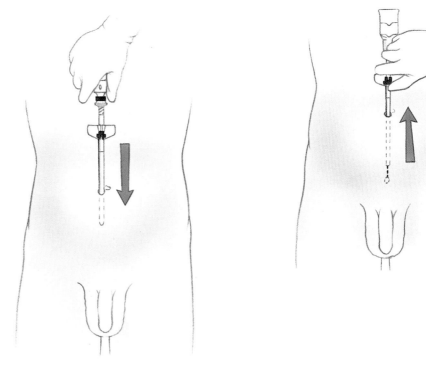

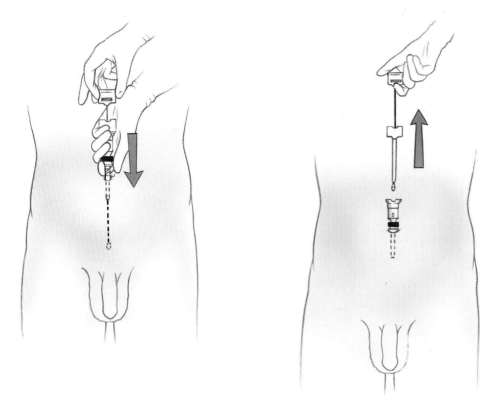

Figure 9.4 (Left)
Advance cannula into space.

Figure 9.5 (Right)
Remove centre rod and obturator.

once this is identified dissection is continued down to the external iliac vessels exposing the direct hernia site. When this is accomplished the dissection is continued superiorly to expose the internal inguinal ring and an indirect sac, if present. Dissection is continued to ensure good exposure around the internal inguinal ring.

If there is a small indirect hernia present this can be dissected away from cord structures; a larger sac, however, is entered anteromedially and severed leaving the distal sac in place. Throughout the dissection care is taken not to puncture the peritoneum as this allows escape of carbon dioxide into the peritoneal space and may result in loss of the operating space. Structural balloons could also be used in creating an operating extraperitoneal space (Figs 9.6–9.9).

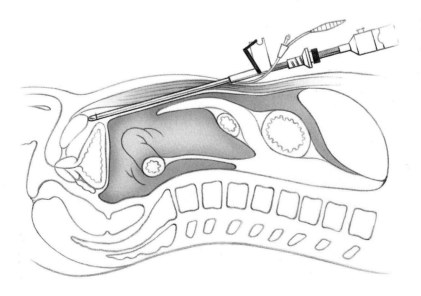

Figure 9.6
Position of the balloon dissector.

Figure 9.7
Balloon inflation.

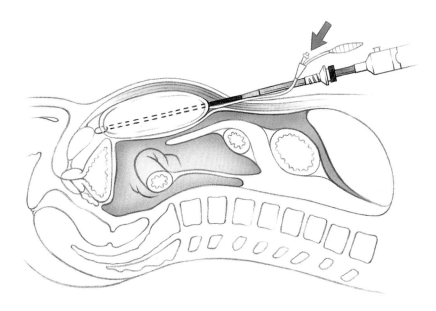

Figure 9.8
Trocar advancement.

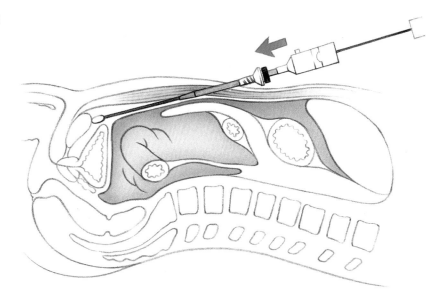

The hernia is repaired by placing a polypropylene mesh (12 × 5 cm) through the 12 mm port and positioning it over the hernial defect. The mesh is secured by initially stapling it to Cooper's ligament and the iliopubic tract; it is then stapled to the transversus abdominus fibres and the lateral border of the rectus abdominus muscle. Bilateral inguinal hernias can be repaired using one large piece of mesh or they can be repaired separately with two pieces of mesh which are joined together in the midline if the defect is large. The extraperitoneal space is then inspected for haemostasis, desufflated, and the skin incisions are then closed. Diathermy use during this procedure should be limited as clearly there may be a risk of thermal injury to structures within the peritoneum such as intestinal loops.

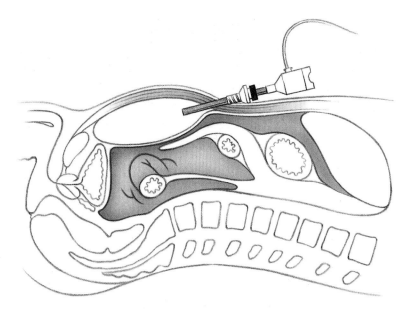

Figure 9.9
Insufflation of the extraperitoneal space.

Discussion

McKernan and Laws have studied the extraperitoneal repair in their initial series of patients [1]. This series consisted of 54 inguinal hernia repairs in 34 patients (29 direct, 22 indirect and 12 bilateral). Two of the patients had their procedures converted from a strictly preperitoneal dissection to an intraperitoneal dissection because of holes being made in the peritoneum during dissection which resulted in a loss of insufflation gas from the extraperitoneal space. Although the follow-up period was short because this was a new procedure, no major complications were noted. Minor complications included orchitis in one patient, and accumulation of fluid in the subcutaneous tissues in three patients. All these complications bar one resolved with conservative management (one patient required aspiration of the fluid collection). There were no recurrences in McKernan and Laws' series and patients returned to work on average 7 days following surgery.

The extraperitoneal hernia repair provides the same benefits that other laparoscopic hernia repairs offer: direct access to the posterior inguinal wall, ability to circumvent scar tissue and adhesions, and a tension-free repair, together with the ease of treating sliding, incarcerated, bilateral and recurrent hernias. The complications of open hernia repair, such as severance of the superficial inguinal nerves, ischaemic orchitis, neuralgia, groin haematomas and infections, are avoided [4].

The extraperitoneal hernia repair is different from the other laparoscopic hernia repairs in that the peritoneal cavity is not intentionally breeched and therefore this eliminates potential problems caused during laparoscopy, such as bowel damage, diathermy injuries and the complications of producing a pneumoperitoneum. Also, by using a total extraperitoneal technique there is no chance of adhesions forming between the prosthetic mesh and bowel. A specific advantage of the extraperitoneal hernia repair has been highlighted recently by the incidence of small bowel obstruction that occurs following a transabdominal preperitoneal repair. This serious and sometimes fatal complication of the laparoscopic transabdominal preperitoneal repair often occurs following the herniation of a knuckle of small bowel between two staples in the peritoneum used to close the peritoneal flaps over the prosthetic mesh [3]. However, the reported cases also include instances where the obstructed bowel simply becomes adherent to the peritoneal defect. Therefore, meticulous technique alone cannot completely avoid this potentially serious complication. The use of an extraperitoneal approach would eliminate this problem as the peritoneum is not incised and therefore no staples are required to close the peritoneum.

The future of safe and effective laparoscopic hernia repair seems to lie in the development of this technique, but for the successful extraperitoneal repair the surgeon must be familiar with laparoscopic procedures. The surgeon should also be proficient in other laparoscopic mesh repairs such as the transabdominal preperitoneal hernia repair. This is often easier than the extraperitoneal approach as the surgeon has the abdominal cavity to manoeuvre in rather than the close confines of the extraperitoneal space. Sound anatomical knowledge of the endoscopic anatomy of the inguinal region is without question the most important factor in safe and effective laparoscopic hernia repair regardless of the technique used (see Chapter 4). The inguinal anatomy as viewed when performing a transabdominal preperitoneal technique tends to be unfamiliar to many surgeons. The anatomy as viewed when performing the extraperitoneal repair is even more unfamiliar because of the different orientation but can be learnt just as well.

Further investigations and long-term follow-up are necessary before conclusions about the procedure's effectiveness and safety can be made. Initial results using this technique have been encouraging and many more surgeons are beginning to turn to laparoscopic extraperitoneal hernia repair as the way forward.

References

1 McKernan JB, Laws HL. Laparoscopic repair of inguinal hernias using a totally extraperitoneal prosthetic approach. *Surg Endosc* 1993; **7**: 26–28.
2 Crist DW, Gadacz TR. Complications of laparoscopic surgery. *Surg Clin North Am* 1993; **73**: 265–289.
3 Corbitt JD. Transabdominal preperitoneal herniorrhaphy. *Surg Laparosc Endosc* 1993; **3**: 328–332.
4 Wantz GE. Complications of inguinal hernia repair. *Surg Clin North Am* 1984; **64**: 287–298.

Chapter 10
Types and safety of synthetic mesh in hernia repair

A. Qureshi, J. Coleman and A. Darzi

Synthetic materials have been evaluated and used in the abdominal wall t6 reinforce [1, 2], replace or substitute for fascia [3] for many years. Mesh fibre sheets have virtually supplanted the use of tantalum mesh, skin or fascia lata grafts as reinforcing materials during inguinal and abdominal wall hernias [4]. Controversy exists concerning the relative advantages of porous or non-porous materials as well as which porous mesh is most appropriate for providing abdominal wall continuity for large abdominal wall defects resulting from trauma or infection [5]. In addition to the above controversies is the surgeon's inherent concern that these foreign bodies will become infected, produce draining sinuses, and require the formidable intervention of complete removal.

A number of techniques have been described including the use of prosthetic materials to assist in the repair. Prosthetic materials have been used to aid in the repair of abdominal wall defects since 1900 [6, 7]. Since then a large number of prosthetic materials have been proposed as the ideal mesh. The criteria necessary for these synthetic materials to be used as prostheses are well established [8, 9]. The criteria include that the prosthetic material:

1 should not be physically modified by tissue fluids;
2 should be chemically inert;
3 should not excite an inflammatory reaction or foreign body reaction;
4 should be non-carcinogenic;
5 should be capable of resisting mechanical strains;
6 should not produce a state of allergy or hypersensitivity;
7 should be capable of being fabricated in the form required;
8 should be capable of being sterilized without alteration of its properties.

While there are a number of prosthetic materials in current use, only a few are commonly utilized. No single material has gained universal acceptance or preference. The ideal prosthesis maintains adequate strength, is incorporated by surrounding tissues and does not stimulate visceral adhesion formation.

Polypropylene mesh (Marlex)

Polypropylene mesh is probably the most common of prosthetic materials used in practice (Figs 10.1 and 10.2). Early studies by Usher have demonstrated that polypropylene mesh is a strong prosthesis [1, 2]. Polypropylene mesh gained widespread use in clinical situations during the Vietnam war [10]. However, long-term complications associated with polypropylene including fistula formation, draining sinuses and mesh extrusion [11, 12] render the prosthesis less than ideal. A commonly ascribed basis for using polypropylene mesh for acute abdominal wall reconstruction is that it may, by virtue of its porosity, allow macromolecular substances to drain from the infected peritoneal cavity. However, there is evidence that the peritoneal cavity is sealed and becomes impermeable to drainage within 12 h even when polypropylene mesh is used [13]. In experimental studies polypropylene mesh does not promote greater peritoneal drainage [14].

Figure 10.1 (Left)
Surgipro^{TM} mesh (Auto Suture, UK)
Figure 10.2 (Right)
Prolene^{TM} knitted polypropylene fibre mesh (Ethicon, UK)

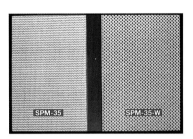 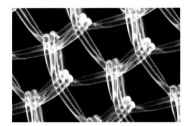

More recent work on the polypropylene mesh has shown that in a 10-year experience in 195 patients with recurrent hernias, the wound infection rate was 2.5% [15]. A 20-year experience by Shulman [16] involving the plug repair of 1402 recurrent hernias and by Lichtenstein [17] repairing over 5000 hernias have found polypropylene mesh to be non-allergenic, non-oncogenic and highly resistant to infection. It serves as an effective and permanent barrier to protrusion through the floor of the inguinal canal.

Polytetrafluoroethylene (PTFE)

This is an expanded microporous polytetrafluorene (filament diameter 140 μm, pore size 500×500 μm) [18]. PTFE produces a slight mononuclear inflammatory cell reaction at the peritoneal surface. The PTFE mesh incorporates into whorls of dense fibrous tissue with numerous fibroblasts, the fibres retaining their position by their fibrous tissue encasement [19]. This fibrous tissue ingrowth among the mesh fibres would indicate that the PTFE mesh is more completely incorporated into the healing wound than other mesh types. Expanded PTFE is used extensively in vascular reconstructive surgery with satisfactory tissue acceptance and it produces minimal foreign body reaction. Jenkins [20] has shown that, when prosthetic materials are used for abdominal reconstruction in rats, the density of adhesions to expanded PTFE was as great as that to polypropylene mesh. This has been corroborated by others [21].

Little information is available concerning peritoneal healing on prosthetic materials, particularly in relationship to the observed clinical complications. Expanded PTFE is able to support a continuous layer of mesothelial cells on the peritoneal surface 4 weeks after implantation [21], but this does not occur with polypropylene or polyglycolic acid meshes as these materials may inhibit mesothelial cell formation because of the chemical nature of the material, or because of the greater inflammatory or foreign body reaction they induce compared with PTFE. In infected wounds, Brown [14] demonstrated that in guinea-pigs expanded PTFE patches stimulated less-dense adhesions than polypropylene mesh 5 days following implantation. However, others [21] have shown that both PTFE and polypropylene meshes induce maximum adhesion formation stimulated by the combination of infection and foreign material. The average 6-year incidence of infection of the PTFE soft tissue patch is 1.8% [18].

Polyglactin (Vicryl)

This is an absorbable suture mesh of moulded polyglactin 910 (Vicryl, measured filament diameter 140 μm, pore size approximately 400×400 μm). Subcutaneous implantation in rats indicates that the absorption of the polyglactin is minimal until about the 42nd postimplantation day. Absorption is essentially complete between 60 and 90 days. In experimental studies performed by Lamb [20], polyglactin mesh maintained satisfactory integrity at 3 weeks for it to be considered as a temporary fascial substitute in patients with abdominal wall defects associated with severe infection. However, at 12 weeks the bursting strength of the polyglactin repair was significantly less than that of non-absorbable prosthetic materials. In addition, 40% of the animals whose wounds were repaired with polyglactin developed ventral hernias.

The evident integrity of the polyglactin mesh at 3 weeks suggests that the material may have some utility in reinforcing fascia during the healing following difficult open hernia repairs. The maintenance of increased wound stability during the initial critical phase of healing with subsequent complete disappearance after primary fascial healing occurs has some theoretical attractiveness. However, the polyglactin mesh may be suitable as a short-term substitute but does not have enough fibrous tissue ingrowth before hydrolysis to render it utilizable without prompt subsequent, overt hernia formation.

Polyglycolic acid

Polyglycolic acid (Dexon) is a synthetic absorbable prosthetic material that can be knitted into sheets of mesh. It is soft, malleable and sterilizable, and is completely absorbed within 90 days after implantation [22]. The precise mechanism of absorption is unclear; however, polyglycolic acid is metabolized into glycolic acid and other carbon intermediates. Phagocytosis by foreign body giant cells occurs at the suture site with deposition of collagen and less tissue reaction than with cotton, silk or catgut. It is eventually excreted by the lungs, kidneys and in the faeces. The rate of absorption is constant and independent of suture diameter. Polyglycolic acid has a high initial tensile strength and maintains this strength for as long as 4 weeks after implantation [23].

Experimental work performed by Law [24] confirmed that the polyglactin mesh initially provided adequate repair while the sutures held the intact mesh, and as the material was hydrolysed the fibrous tissue laid down was insufficient to maintain the integrity of the abdominal wall. Although no overt hernias were seen, the site of the implanted polyglactin mesh bulged in the region of the repair thus representing an area of weakness and a potential site for wound failure. When the polyglactin mesh is used to buttress wounds closed under tension rather than to repair abdominal wall defects, results are superior [25]. Since the mesh is absorbed by 90 days after implantation, the untoward late complications associated with prosthetic materials are avoided.

Conclusion

It has been stated that the 'ideal' prosthetic material should be chemically inert, non-carcinogenic, capable of resisting mechanical stress, capable of being fabricated in the form required and sterilizable, yet not be physically modified by tissue fluids, excite inflammatory or foreign body tissue reaction or induce a state of allergy or hypersensitivity. However, currently available prostheses fall short of this goal.

The absorbable prostheses available maintain sufficient strength for only a short period of time, while long-term support is inadequate. However, long-term complications associated with the non-absorbable prostheses are avoided. Adhesion formation is also significantly less compared with the non-absorbable prostheses [20]. Nonetheless, the use of the absorbable prosthetic mesh may be limited to short-term substitute only.

PTFE mesh evaluated previously as a macroporous mesh was found to be associated with unsatisfactory infection rates compared with polypropylene mesh used for hernia repair wounds in humans [26]. More recent studies, however, indicate that both microporous PTFE mesh and polypropylene mesh showed no significant difference in infection rates or in inflammatory cell infiltrates [19]. Crimping and folding are associated with fluid accumulation and hence increased infection rates [4].

In conclusion, whereas the absorbable prostheses provide the best long-term protection against infection and adhesions, the non-absorbable prostheses are superior for permanent abdominal wall replacement.

References

1 Usher FC, Gannon JP. Marlex mesh, a new plastic mesh for replacing tissue defects. *Arch Surg* 1959; **78**: 131–137.
2 Usher FC, Fries JG, Ochsner JL, Tuttle LLD. Marlex mesh—a new plastic mesh for replacing tissue defects. II Clinical studies. *Arch Surg* 1959; **78**: 138–145.
3 Ogilvie WH. The late complications of abdominal war wounds. *Lancet* 1940; **ii**: 253–256.
4 Smith RS. The use of prosthetic materials in the repair of hernias. *Surg Clin North Am* 1971; **51**: 1387–1389.
5 Goris RJA. Ogilvie's method applied to infected wound disruption. *Arch Surg* 1980; **115**: 1103–1107.
6 Witzel O. Über den verschluss von bauchwunden und bruchphorten durch versenkte silver-drahtnetze (Einheilung von filigranpelotten). *Centralbl Chir* 1990; **27**: 257–260.
7 Goepel R. Ueber die verschliessung von bruchphorten durch einheilung gelflochtener, fertiger silberdrahtnetze (silberdrahtpelotten). *Verh Dsch Ges Chir* 1990; **29**: 174–177.
8 Cumberland VH. A preliminary report on the use of prefabricated nylon weave in the repair of ventral hernia. *Med J Aust* 1952; **1**: 143–144.
9 Scales JT. Tissue reactions to synthetic materials. *Proc R Soc Med* 1953; **46**: 647–652.
10 Schmitt HJ, Grinnan LB. Use of Marlex mesh in infected abdominal war wounds. *Am J Surg* 1967; **113**: 825–828.

11 Voyles CR, Richardson JD, Bland KI, Tobin GR, Flint LM, Polk HC. Emergency abdominal wall reconstruction with polypropylene mesh. *Ann urg* 1981; **194** 219–223.

12 Stone HH, Fabian TC, Turkleson ML, Jurkiewicz MJ. Management of acute full thickness losses of the abdominal wall due to infection. *Ann Surg* 1981; **193**: 612–618.

13 Boyd WC. Use of Marlex mesh in acute loss of the abdominal wall due to infection. *Surg Gynaecol Obstet* 1977; **144**: 251–252.

14 Brown GL, Richardson JD, Malangoni MA, Tobin GR, Ackerman D, Polk HC. Comparison of prosthetic materials for abdominal wall reconstruction in the presence of contamination and infection. *Ann Surg* 1985; **201**: 705–711.

15 Nyhus LM, Pollak R, Bombeck CT *et al.* The preperitoneal approach and prosthetic buttress repair for recurrent hernia: The evolution of a technique. *Ann Surg* 1988; **208**: 733.

16 Shulman AG, Amid PK, Lichtenstein IL. The 'plug' repair of 1402 recurrent inguinal hernias. 20 year experience. *Arch Surg* 1990; **125**(2): 265–267.

17 Lichtenstein IL, Shulman AG, Amid PK. Use of mesh to prevent recurrent hernias. *Postgrad Med* 1990; **87**: 155–158.

18 GORE-TEX *Soft Tissue Patch Technical Bulletin. Technical Considerations in Hernia Repair*. WL Gore & Associates, Inc., 1989.

19 Lamb JP, Vitale T, Kaminski DL. Comparative evaluation of synthetic meshes used for abdominal wall replacement. *Surgery* 1983; **93**: 643–648.

20 Jenkins SD, Klamer TW, Parteka JJ, Condon RE. A comparison of prosthetic materials used to repair abdominal wall defects. *Surgery* 1983; **94**: 392–398.

21 Law NW, Ellis H. Adhesion formation and peritoneal healing on prosthetic materials. *Clin Materials* 1988; **3**: 95–101.

22 Katz AR, Turner AJ. Evaluation of tensile and absorption properties of polyglycolic acid sutures. *Surg Gynaecol Obstet* 1970; **131**: 701–716.

23 Hermann JB, Kelly RJ, Higgins GA. Polyglycolic acid sutures: Laboratory and clinical evaluation of a new absorbable suture material. *Arch Surg* 1974; **100**: 486–490.

24 Law NW. A comparison of polypropylene mesh, expanded polytetrafluoroethylene patch and polyglycolic acid mesh for the repair of experimental abdominal wall defects. *Acta Chir Scand* 1990; **156**: 759–762.

25 Marmon LM, Vinocur CD, Staniford SB, Wagner CW, Dunn JM, Weintraub WH. Evaluation of absorbable polyglycolic acid mesh as a wound support. *J Ped Surg* 1985; **20**: 737–742.

26 Gibson LD, Stafford CE. Synthetic mesh repair of abdominal wall defects. *Am Surg* 1964; **30**: 481–486.

Further reading

Arnaud JP, Eloy R, Adloff M, Grenier JF. Critical evaluation of prosthetic materials in repair of adbominal wall hernias. *Am J Surg* 1977; **133**: 338–345.

Hamer-Hodges DW, Scott NB. Replacement of an abdominal wall defect using expanded PTFE sheet (GORE-TEX). *J R Coll Surg Edinb* 1985; **30**: 65–67.

Law NW, Ellis H. Preliminary results for the repair of difficult recurrent inguinal hernias using expanded PTFE patch. *Acta Chir Scand* 1990; **156**: 609–612.

Law NW, Ellis H. A comparison of polypropylene mesh and expanded polytetrafluoroethylene patch for the repair of contaminated abdominal wall defects—an experimental study. *Surgery* 1991; **109**: 652–655.

Chapter 11

Balloon-assisted extraperitoneal laparoscopic hernia repair

A.K. Chin, F.H. Moll and M.B. McColl

Totally extraperitoneal laparoscopic herniorrhaphy addresses some of the perceived disadvantages of transabdominal preperitoneal laparoscopic hernia repair: namely, violation of the peritoneal cavity and the requirement for general anaesthesia [1]. Incision and subsequent repair of the peritoneum raises concerns about potential postoperative adhesion formation. Conversion of an open hernia repair performed with local anaesthesia to a laparoscopic procedure conducted under general anaesthesia offers the patient shortened convalescence at an associated cost of increased anaesthetic morbidity. The use of pneumoperitoneum during laparoscopic hernia repair also contributes to untoward physiological side-effects, including cardiac arrhythmias [2, 3], acidosis [4, 5], subcutaneous emphysema and gas embolism [6].

Over the past several years, multiple authors have described their techniques for development of an extraperitoneal cavity and mesh repair of inguinal hernias [7–10]. McKernan [7, 9] describes the use of a periumbilical incision to dissect through the fascia and rectus muscle to the preperitoneal space. A 10 mm operating laparoscope with a 5 mm blunt probe inserted through the working channel is advanced through the incision and used to form an extraperitoneal tunnel to the symphysis pubis. Two trocars are inserted into the tunnel, and a suction device and laparoscopic grasper are advanced through the ports and used to complete the dissection of the preperitoneal cavity. Arregui *et al.* [10] use a combined extra- and intra-abdominal approach, with transperitoneal endoscopic monitoring of the extraperitoneal dissection process. A 5 mm trocar is inserted in the anterior axillary line at the level of the umbilicus, and introduced into the preperitoneal space. Blunt dissection is used to prepare the preperitoneal cavity.

Blunt dissection of the preperitoneal space using manual displacement of the peritoneum has several disadvantages. Firstly, the technique is cumbersome, requiring multiple strokes of the blunt probe to form an adequate cavity size. Secondly, the anatomical landmarks are difficult to appreciate, owing to dissection in the preperitoneal fat layer. Displacement of the peritoneum within this layer occurs slowly, and strands of fat and connective tissue hang down from the ceiling of the cavity, obscuring visualization and identification of pertinent structures. Thirdly, multiple probing with a 5 mm instrument increases the potential for peritoneal perforation and tissue disruption. Peritoneal perforation leads to intra-abdominal insufflation upon preperitoneal gas instillation, ruling out the use of local or regional anaesthesia. Tissue disruption and small vessel avulsion result in bleeding within the extraperitoneal cavity, further obscuring surgical visualization.

We propose the use of a balloon cannula to assist in the preperitoneal dissection process. The cannula has a balloon attached to its distal end, and accommodates a 10 mm laparoscope within its central lumen. The device is inserted via a periumbilical incision, advanced to the symphysis pubis within the extraperitoneal plane, and inflated to create a preperitoneal working cavity. A laparoscope resides within the balloon during inflation, permitting direct visualisation of the dissection process. This allows the surgeon to verify correct preperitoneal placement of the cannula during balloon dissection, and it avoids inadvertent avulsion of blood vessels which may occur with blind dissection techniques. Balloon inflation is accomplished using a squeeze bulb; air inflation yields a cushioned, gentle dissection, due to the compressibility of air. Abrupt inflation volume changes which may occur with fluid injection into the balloon and lead to peritoneal disruption are moderated with air inflation. Air inflation also facilitates balloon deflation and cannula removal following dissection.

Device description

Two versions of the dissection balloon cannula have been developed. The first version incorporates a spherical, elastomeric balloon which forms a central cavity useful for unilateral groin dissection or access into the space of Retzius and the bladder neck. The second version uses a kidney-shaped, relatively inelastic balloon to achieve lateral dissection upon balloon inflation. This version is designed to develop the broad preperitoneal cavity required for bilateral hernia repair. Both versions are manufactured and distributed by Origin Medsystems, Menlo Park, California, USA. The spherical balloon cannula (Preperitoneal Distention Balloon: PDB™) is depicted in Fig. 11.1. The balloon cannula consists of an inflation tube with an attached spherical silicone rubber balloon. The selected inflation tube length allows the tip of an inserted laparoscope to extend into the cavity of the balloon. A proximal valve body houses a one-way valve for balloon inflation and a desufflation button which opens a flapper valve. A removable obturator is inserted through the cannula to provide blunt

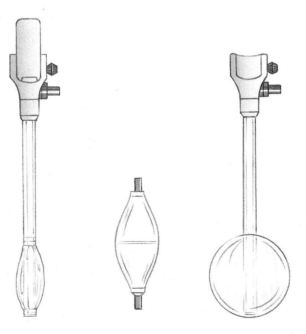

Figure 11.1
The components of the spherical balloon dissection cannula. The elastomeric balloon inflates in a spherical fashion, as illustrated.

inner support for the balloon during cannula advancement through the preperitoneal tissue. Balloon inflation is performed by means of a rubber inflation bulb as shown.

The bilateral balloon dissection cannula (Preperitoneal Distention Balloon 2) is illustrated in Fig. 11.2. This cannula utilizes a relatively inelastic balloon for preperitoneal dissection. The uninflated balloon is rolled up against the inflation tube and encased by a perforated outer sheath. Initial inflation with the inflation bulb splits the outer sheath and releases the balloon; subsequent balloon inflation forms a broad cavity extending laterally in both directions within the preperitoneal space.

Following extraperitoneal cavity formation, the dissected space is distended by means of gas insufflation. The balloon dissection cannula is removed, and a blunt-tipped balloon trocar is used to seal the entrance to the preperitoneal space. The blunt-tipped trocar (Fig. 11.3) consists of a sleeve with a small distal silicone rubber balloon that

Figure 11.2

The bilateral balloon dissection cannula has a perforated sheath that encases a relatively inelastic plastic balloon which inflates to a kidney-shaped configuration.

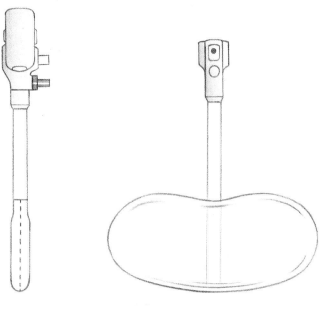

Figure 11.3

The blunt tip balloon trocar is used to seal the entrance tract and allow insufflation into the preperitoneal space.

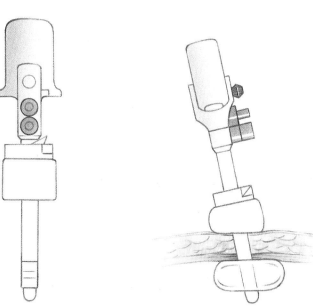

is inflated to contact the sides of the tunnel leading to the preperitoneal cavity. A locking collar with a foam cuff is brought down to the skin surface, gently compressing the abdominal tissue to form a leak-tight seal. The valve body of the blunt-tipped trocar houses a balloon inflation port, an insufflation port, a flapper valve, and built-in convertors that accommodate scope and instrument sizes between 3 and 10 mm.

Technique

Balloon-assisted preparation of the preperitoneal space consists of four steps:

1 Periumbilical incision and dissection to the correct plane for cannula insertion.
2 Cannula advancement and balloon inflation.
3 Blunt-tipped trocar placement and preperitoneal gas insufflation.
4 Isolation of the anatomical landmarks in the preperitoneal space.

The remainder of the preperitoneal herniorrhaphy procedure proceeds in the usual fashion, with the placement of secondary instrument ports, hernia sac dissection, and mesh placement.

Periumbilical dissection

A 15 mm skin incision is made. The skin incision may be infraumbilical, for cosmetic indications, or paramedian, at the level of the umbilicus. The entrance tract should be 1–2 cm lateral of midline, regardless of the initial skin incision. For a unilateral hernia repair, an ipsilateral placement of the insertion tract is used; for a bilateral repair, the insertion tract may be on either side of the midline. In the case of an infraumbilical incision, the skin is retracted laterally to permit entrance tract dissection in a paramedian location. Following skin incision, the subcutaneous tissue is cleared from the underlying fascial layer, using blunt or electrocautery dissection. The first fascial layer, the anterior rectus sheath, is incised sharply for a length of 15 mm (Fig. 11.4).

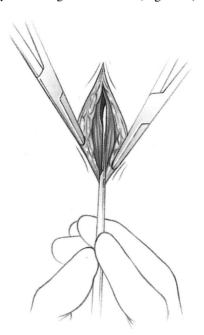

Figure 11.4
The cannula insertion incision. The skin is incised and the subcutaneous fat is dissected away to expose the anterior rectus sheath, which is sharply incised to reveal the rectus muscle.

The exposed rectus muscle is spread apart, using a pair of curved or straight haemostatic clamps, until the surface of the posterior rectus sheath comes into view. A gloved finger is inserted on top of the posterior rectus sheath, and advanced inferiorly in the direction of the symphysis pubis, to initiate the tract for dissection balloon cannula placement (Fig. 11.5). Following dissection, the entrance tract should fit loosely around the inserted finger, to adequately accommodate advancement of the balloon cannula.

Figure 11.5

Following incision of the anterior rectus sheath and spreading of the rectus muscle, a gloved finger is used to initiate a tract directly on top of the posterior rectus sheath.

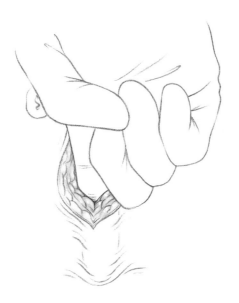

Cannula advancement and balloon inflation

After checking to ensure that the obturator is fully seated within the cannula, the dissection balloon cannula is introduced into the dissected paramedian tract, and placed directly against the posterior rectus sheath. While keeping the cannula parallel to the plane of the abdominal wall, the cannula is gently advanced to the symphysis pubis, with a twisting motion of the device applied to aid its progression through the preperitoneal tissue. As the cannula is advanced towards the symphysis, care should be taken not to angle the cannula anteriorly, into the rectus muscle, or posteriorly, causing entry into the abdominal cavity. Initially, the dissection balloon cannula will lie on top of the posterior rectus sheath. As the cannula is advanced inferiorly past the arcuate line, the posterior rectus sheath ends, automatically locating the cannula in the preperitoneal space. Arrival of the cannula tip at the symphysis pubis may be verified by external palpation. Following full cannula insertion, the obturator is removed and replaced with the laparoscope. The inflation bulb is used to inflate the balloon. After several compressions of the inflation bulb, the laparoscope may be advanced into the balloon cavity to view the progress of the dissection and the developing anatomical landmarks. Forty compressions with the inflation bulb correspond to approximately a 750 ml cavity, which is generally an adequate sized operating cavity. Upon completion of balloon dissection, the laparoscope is removed from the cannula, and the desufflation button depressed to deflate the balloon. The dissection balloon cannula is removed from the insertion tract. Insertion and inflation of the balloon cannula are depicted in Fig. 11.6, as well as blunt-tipped trocar placement, as described below.

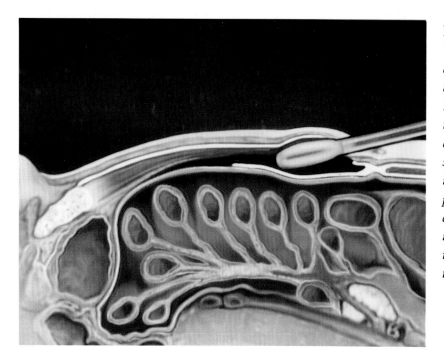

Figure 11.6
The sequence of events in cannula advancement and balloon dissection. (a) The Balloon cannula is introduced into the insertion tract. (b) The cannula is advanced to the symphysis pubis. (c) The balloon is inflated with the laparoscope positioned within the balloon cavity. (d) The balloon cannula is removed and the blunt tip trocar used to seal the insertion tract for gas insufflation.

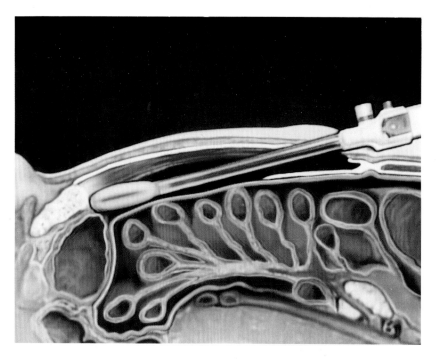

Figure 11.6b

Figure 11.6c

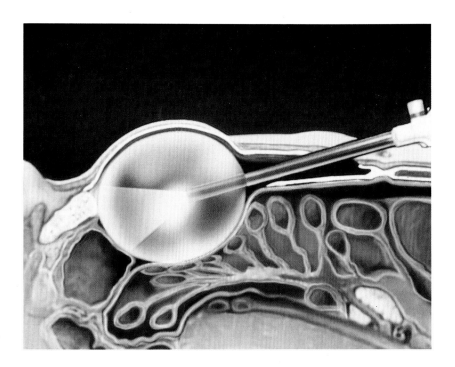

Figure 11.6d

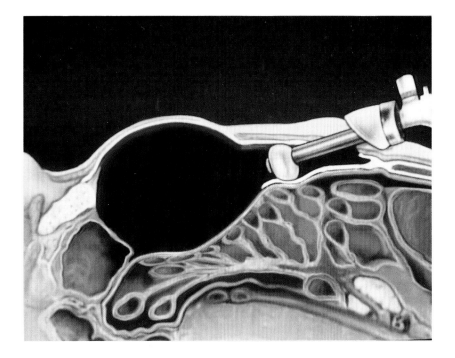

Blunt-tipped trocar placement and preperitoneal gas insufflation

The blunt-tipped trocar is inserted into the entrance tract and the distal balloon is inflated with 25 ml of air or 20 ml of saline. The locking collar is placed against the skin, compressing the foam cuff slightly to provide a reliable gas-tight seal. The blunt obturator is removed from the trocar and gas insufflation introduced into the preperitoneal space, to a pressure of 10–12 mmHg. The laparoscope is introduced via the blunt-tipped trocar, and the secondary trocar ports placed in the desired locations. Both ancillary ports are often placed in the midline: one midway between the umbilicus and the symphysis pubis, and the other 1–2 cm above the symphysis pubis [9].

Isolation of the anatomical landmarks in the preperitoneal space

The most visible anatomical landmark following preperitoneal balloon dissection is Cooper's ligament, which appears as a white ridge extending laterally from the pubic tubercle in the midline (Fig. 11.7). External digital pressure applied to the midline above the symphysis pubis will cause a visible depression inside the preperitoneal cavity, and assist in giving the surgeon a point of orientation. In obese patients, blunt dissection of the preperitoneal fat away from Cooper's ligament will help delineate this initial landmark. Proceeding laterally along Cooper's ligament, the iliac vessels will come into view; these may be followed up to the origin of the epigastric vessels, which in turn give the location of the internal inguinal ring. The internal ring lies lateral to the epigastric vessels, which may be seen coursing vertically on the preperitoneal pelvic floor.

Identification of the internal inguinal ring allows the surgeon to proceed with dissection of the indirect hernial sac and skeletonization of the cord structures. Hernial sac delineation is more difficult in the preperitoneal space as compared with the transabdominal approach, as no obvious indirect hernial defect may be appreciated in the extraperitoneal tissue. Careful dissection is required to isolate the sac; however, application of a systematic approach as outlined above will generally allow the surgeon to complete the repair in an expedient fashion.

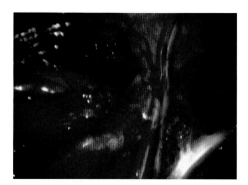

Figure 11.7
View of the balloon-dissected preperitoneal space, with colour enhancements added to point out Cooper's ligament (in white) and the iliac vessels (in red and blue).

Clinical use

Hernia repair

During the past year, balloon-assisted preperitoneal dissection has been utilized in over 1100 patients undergoing total preperitoneal laparoscopic hernia repair. Balloon dissection has simplified preperitoneal cavity preparation, with no reported incidence of epigastric vessel injury or avulsion. Technique issues which have been noted include the following:

1 *Correct preparation of the balloon cannula insertion tract is essential to preperitoneal cavity formation.* The surgeon should verify that the cannula is inserted directly on top of the posterior rectus sheath at the incision site. Adequate incision of the skin and anterior rectus sheath is necessary to avoid difficult advancement of the balloon cannula.

2 *Advancement of the cannula should proceed in a plane parallel with the abdominal wall.* If the cannula is angled upward during advancement, the balloon will become embedded in the rectus muscle. Balloon inflation may result in separation of the epigastric vessels from the overlying muscle, causing them to be suspended in the centre of the preperitoneal cavity, hindering instrument movement and mesh placement. The suspended vessels may need to be ligated and divided to provide an unobstructed approach for hernia sac dissection. Inflation of the balloon within the body of the rectus muscle may also result in blood oozing into the surgical field, due to disruption of minute vessels within the muscle. If the balloon cannula is angled downward during advancement, the cannula tip may puncture through the peritoneum inferior to the arcuate line, where the tough posterior rectus sheath is no longer present to redirect the cannula from intra-abdominal entry. Peritoneal puncture leads to general abdominal insufflation upon gas infusion into the preperitoneal space, rendering it difficult to perform the surgery under local or regional anaesthesia.

3 *Prior peritoneal incision and dissection result in difficult formation of the preperitoneal cavity.* Fibrosis and adhesion of the peritoneum to preperitoneal tissue makes it prone to tearing upon dissection by either balloon inflation or blunt instrument displacement. This has been experienced with recurrent laparoscopic hernia repair and prior bladder surgery which requires dissection of the peritoneum in the pelvic area. On the other hand, extraperitoneal balloon dissection functions well in laparoscopic repair of recurrent inguinal hernia, where the initial repair was performed as an open procedure. In this situation, the preperitoneal plane is relatively undisturbed by the first procedure, and widespread fibrosis is avoided.

Laparoscopic total preperitoneal hernia repair may be performed without gas insufflation, using a mechanical lift system (Fig. 11.8) to support the abdominal wall while displacing the dissected peritoneum downwards with a laparoscopic retractor. Balloon dissection of the preperitoneal space is accomplished, followed by insertion

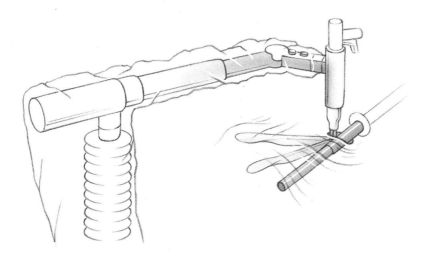

Figure 11.8
The mechanical lift system used for gasless laparoscopy. A fan retractor used to retract tissue is hoisted by a motorized lifting arm.

of a fan retractor to displace the abdominal wall. Newman *et al.* [11] describe the use of this mechanical system to perform transabdominal laparoscopic herniorrhaphy. G. Ferzli (personal communication) has applied the system to total preperitoneal laparoscopic hernia repair, coupled with balloon dissection of the working space, under local anaesthesia. A gasless approach is advantageous for two reasons. Firstly, it allows total preperitoneal procedures to be conducted under local or regional anaesthesia in the event of peritoneal perforation, since intra-abdominal insufflation does not occur. Secondly, it enables multiple, conventional surgical instruments to be applied in laparoscopic procedures, increasing operative dexterity and control [12].

Lymphadenectomy

The balloon cannula has been applied to extraperitoneal laparoscopic resection of lymph nodes residing along the obturator and iliac vessels in pelvic staging procedures conducted particularly for prostatic carcinoma. The spherical, elastomeric balloon cannula is generally used for this procedure, since a central cavity is required, without substantial lateral extension of the extraperitoneal space. The cannula insertion site is the identical one used for laparoscopic preperitoneal hernia repair. Two ancillary instrument ports are inserted—a 10 mm port and a 5 mm port—in locations similar to those described above for bilateral hernia repair. A right-angled haemostatic clip applier [13] may be introduced via the 10 mm port to assist with ductal ligation during nodal resection. The extraperitoneal approach allows the staging procedure to be performed under restricted anaesthesia use.

Incontinence surgery

Bladder neck suspension techniques such as the Burch procedure [14] may be performed in the preperitoneal space, without the need for transabdominal laparoscopic instrumentation and general anaesthesia. A spherical, elastomeric balloon cannula is applied via a periumbilical incision to dissect a midline cavity incorporating the bladder neck region. The spherical balloon opens the space of Retzius, and allows bilateral periurethral sutures to be placed. Anchoring of these respective sutures in Cooper's ligament results in suspension of the bladder neck and completion of the procedure.

Discussion

Balloon-assisted preparation of the extraperitoneal cavity facilitates a tedious part of the total preperitoneal laparoscopic herniorrhaphy procedure: that is, dissection of the preperitoneal working space and identification of important anatomical landmarks. It does so by employing soft balloon dissection under direct visual scrutiny. Endoscopic visualization during the dissection process imparts control over cannula positioning, the rate of tissue displacement, and the final cavity size. It allows the determination of correct cannula placement in the preperitoneal cavity, and in the event of an initial puncture through the peritoneum it prevents the blind continuation of balloon inflation with extended peritoneal rupture as a result. Air inflation of the dissection balloon teases apart tissue layers in a cushioned manner. Air inflation also avoids the inconvenience and added weight applied with saline inflation of a 750 ml balloon. No concerns exist regarding the possibility of gas embolism upon balloon rupture, since the open channel formed by the space between the cannula and the surrounding tissue tunnel instantaneously equalizes the pressure between the preperitoneal cavity and the outside atmosphere.

The attractiveness of total preperitoneal laparoscopic hernia repair in terms of decreased postoperative recovery period, preservation of an intact peritoneum, and potential use of local and regional anaesthesia, has previously been diminished by the increased difficulty of working cavity formation and structure identification in the extraperitoneal space. The visual balloon cannula addresses these concerns, and decreases the learning curve associated with the adoption of total preperitoneal endoscopy. The utility of this approach extends to other applications, such as lymphadenectomy and bladder neck suspension. The ability to maintain the balloon-formed preperitoneal space with a mechanical lifting system adds another dimension to the procedure. A gasless approach to preperitoneal surgery relaxes the constraints on specific laparoscopic instrumentation, and allows conventional open surgical instruments to be applied. This approach may enable more complicated pre-peritoneal and retroperitoneal techniques to be developed.

Summary

Simple balloon dissection of the extraperitoneal space has appeared to simplify the procedure of total preperitoneal laparoscopic herniorrhaphy. The next level of progression, including gasless retraction techniques and more sophisticated multilobular balloon structures, is already in development. Continued work in these areas will hopefully expand the boundaries of the field of less invasive surgery.

References

1 Macintyre IMC. Laparoscopic herniorrhaphy. *Br J Surg* 1992; **79**: 1123–1124.

2 Myles PS. Bradyarrhythmias and laparoscopy: A prospective study of heart rate changes with laparoscopy. *Aust NZ Obstet Gynaecol* 1991; **31**: 171–173.

3 Motew M, Ivankovich AD, Bieniarz J *et al*. Cardiovascular effects and acid–base and blood gas changes during laparoscopy. *Am J Obstet Gynecol* 1973; **115**: 1002–1011.

4 Holzman M, Sharp K, Richards W. Hypercarbia during carbon dioxide gas insufflation for therapeutic laparoscopy: A note of caution. *Surg Laparosc Endosc* 1992; **2**(1): 11–14.

5 Kent RB III. Subcutaneous emphysema and hypercarbia following laparoscopic cholecystectomy. *Arch Surg* 1991; **126**: 1154–1156.

6 Clark CC, Weeks DB, Gusdon JP. Venous carbon dioxide embolism during laparoscopy. *Anesth Analg* 1977; **56**: 650–652.

7 McKernan JB. Laparoscopic preperitoneal prosthetic repair of inguinal hernias. *Surg Rounds* **1992**; **15**(7): 597–610.

8 Ferzli GS, Massaad A, Sysarz FA III *et al*. A study of 101 patients treated with extraperitoneal endoscopic laparoscopic herniorrhaphy. *Am Surg* 1993; **59**: 707–708.

9 McKernan JB, Laws HL. Laparoscopic repair of inguinal hernias using a totally extraperitoneal prosthetic approach. *Surg Endosc* 1993; **7**: 26–28.

10 Arregui ME, Navarette J, Davis CJ *et al*. Laparoscopic inguinal herniorrhaphy. *Surg Clin North Am* 1993; **73**(3): 513–527.

11 Newman L III, Luke JP, Ruben DM, Eubanks S. Laparoscopic herniorrhaphy without pneumoperitoneum. *Surg Laparosc Endosc* 1993; **3**(3): 213–215.

12 Chin AK, Moll FH, McColl MB, Reich H. Mechanical peritoneal retraction as a replacement for carbon dioxide pneumoperitoneum. *J Am Assoc Gynecol Laparosc* 1993; **1**(1): 62–66.

13 Chin AK, Moll FH, McColl MB. Novel technique and instrumentation for laparoscopic application of hemostatic clips. *J Am Assoc Gynecol Laparosc* 1994; **1**(2): 150–153.

14 Underwood LR, Smith ML Jr. Minimally invasive management of genuine urinary stress incontinence. *AAGL 22nd Annual Meeting 1993* (abstract).

Chapter 12
Endoscopic sutured repair

A. Qureshi, A. Leahy and H. Osborne

Introduction

The importance of closure of the internal inguinal ring during repair of inguinal hernias was stressed in 1887 by Marcy [1] who described inguinal hernia repair by simple closure of the internal inguinal ring with excision of the sac through an intra-abdominal approach. This method was later modified by LaRoque [2] who suggested that the intra-abdominal route for repair of inguinal and femoral hernia provided an accurate diagnosis and reduced trauma to vital structures at the deep ring. Coincidental repair of indirect inguinal hernias during unrelated laparotomy for other diseases was recognized by Andrews [3] who suggested that this method was a far more effective repair compared with other repairs at the time. Herniotomy on its own has been used for inguinal hernia repair in infants and young adults up to the age of 18 years with impressive results [4]. With the availability of laparoscopic technology it is possible to perform a similar procedure in a select group of patients. Ger in 1982 demonstrated that simple closure of the neck of the sac of abdominal wall hernias in adults was an effective method in the management of these hernias [5]. With the recent advancements in technology of instrumentation and improvement in the laparoscopic skill of the surgeon, laparoscopic closure of the neck of the sac is now possible.

Patients

Between August 1990 and September 1992, 77 healthy males with a mean age of 31.4 years (range 18–58 years) presented with an indirect inguinal hernia. Four patients had bilateral hernias. Sixty-two patients were offered one of two different laparoscopic inguinal hernia repairs, and 15 patients underwent a traditional Bassini repair. Choice of operation depended on the preference of the operating surgeon. Patient details are given in Table 12.1.

Methods

Laparoscopic hernia repairs

Under general endotracheal anaesthesia, with the patient flat upon the table, a pneumoperitoneum was induced with carbon dioxide administered via a Veress needle. A 0° laparoscope was introduced through a 10 mm trocar placed in the infraumbilical position. An indirect inguinal hernia was confirmed in all cases by direct vision of a patent internal ring and by visualization and palpation of an inguinal swelling

	Laparoscopic repair			
	Purse-string	External needle	Bassini repair
No. of hernias	30	36	15
% male	100	100	100
Mean age (years)	29.3±12.2	39.5±13.2	32.7±16.4
Anaesthesia time (min)	106.5±41.7	82.8±34.1	72.3±28.2
Pain scale	1.6±0.9	2.1±1.1	5.4±1.6†
Complications	1	0	3*
Postop. stay (days)	1.7±0.5	1.8±0.6	3.7±2.0†
Recurrence	1	1	0

*$P<0.01$.
†$P<0.001$.

Table 12.1
Comparison of laparoscopic and Bassini inguinal hernia repairs.

secondary to distension of the hernial sac with carbon dioxide. A further two 5 mm trocars were inserted in the right and left hypochondrium respectively.

Purse-string closure of internal ring. Through one of the 5 mm trocars a needle holder with a 2/0 silk suture on a 30 mm straight taper-cut needle was inserted, while through the other a grasping forceps was inserted. The internal ring was obliterated by a double purse-string technique. Figure 12.1 demonstrates clearly the vas deferens and the testicular vessels. The neck of the hernial sac was closed by insertion of a purse-string suture around the neck thus approximating the sides of the internal ring. This was reinforced by insertion of a second purse-string suture which had the effect of inverting the first (Fig. 12.2). In all cases, damage to the

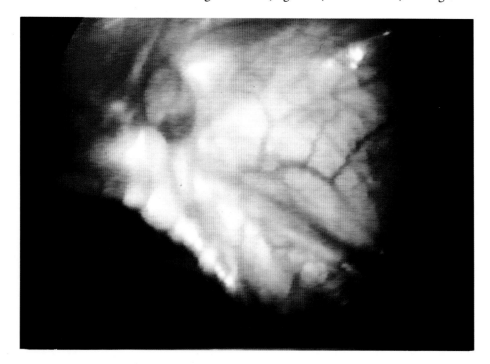

Figure 12.1
View of internal ring demonstrating the vas deferens and testicular vessels.

Figure 12.2
View of internal ring following closure by insertion of purse-string suture.

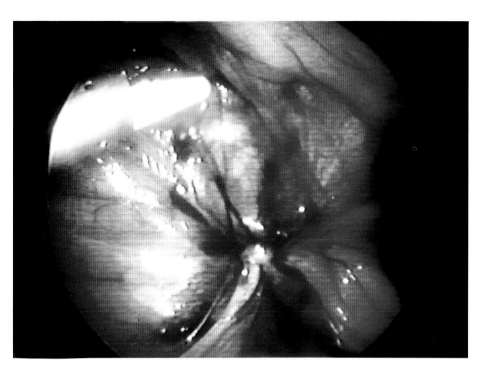

spermatic cord and inferior epigastric vessels was avoided by direct visualization of these structures.

External needle closure of the internal ring. An alternative technique allows for closure of the deep ring by an externally introduced needle guided under laparoscopic control.

The deep inguinal ring was identified and circumcised to disconnect the sac from the deep ring. The vas deferens, testicular vessels and inferior epigastric vessels are easily visualized to avoid any injury. An external hollow needle specially constructed with a bend at the end was passed through the anterior abdominal wall superior and lateral to the deep ring [6]. The needle was handled from the outside and picked up the upper followed by the lower peritoneal flaps. The central trocar of the needle was removed, and a no. 1 nylon suture was passed through the hollow needle, picked up using a grasper and brought out through one of the ports. The point of the needle was retracted to release both upper and lower peritoneal flaps and again the nylon suture material was picked up and brought out through the same port as before. An extracorporeal knot was tied and pushed down to the level of the deep ring [7]. This was repeated three times to secure the knot in place. Several interrupted knots were placed approximately 0.5 cm apart, allowing adequate and complete closure of the deep inguinal ring.

Bassini repair

Under general endotracheal anaesthesia, with the patient flat upon the table, a suprainguinal incision was made and the external oblique aponeurosis exposed. This was incised and split along its fibres extending laterally from the deep ring and medially to the superficial ring. The edges of the peritoneal sac were identified within the cord and cleared as far back as the internal ring. After the sac had been opened and the contents inspected and replaced, the sac was ligated with a strong transfixation suture. The sac was then excised distal to the transfixation suture. After the sac had been removed, the lower border of the conjoint muscles and tendon were approximated, using 5–6 interrupted 2/0 Prolene sutures at 1 cm intervals, to the upturned edge of the inguinal ligament. A Tanner slide, involving a 2 cm vertical incision on the anterior rectus sheath 2.5 cm above the repair, was added to overcome tension.

The operative time, pain experienced at 24 h (on a visual analogue pain scale where 0 represents no pain and 10 is the worst imaginable pain), complications, postoperative stay and recurrence were compared between the two groups of patients. Data are expressed as mean ± standard deviation; Student's t test for unpaired observations and the χ^2 test were used for statistical analysis. $P<0.05$ was considered significant.

Results

Laparoscopic purse-string herniorraphy was successful in all 30 patients in whom it was attempted and laparoscopic external needle herniorraphy in another 36 patients. A Bassini repair was carried out in 15 patients. In three patients it was necessary to dissect free the greater omentum from the hernial sac prior to initiation of laparoscopic hernial sac closure. All patients were male. The results are summarised in Table 12.1.

The mean age of the patients undergoing laparoscopic purse-string closure was 29.3±12.2 years compared with 39.5±13.2 years for the laparoscopic external needle closure group and 32.7±16.4 years for the Bassini group. The mean anaesthetic time for the laparoscopic purse-string group was 106.5±41.7 min compared with 82.8±34.1 min for the laparoscopic external needle closure group and 72.3±28.2 min for the Bassini repair ($P<0.01$). The laparoscopic purse-string group recorded a mean pain measurement of 1.6±0.9 at 24 h compared with 2.1±1.1 for the laparoscopic external needle closure group and 5.4±1.6 for the Bassini herniorraphy group, on the visual analogue pain scale ($P<0.001$). There was one case of postoperative urinary retention in the laparoscopic purse-string group; one wound infection and two cases of postoperative urinary retention requiring catheterization occurred in the Bassini group.

At a mean follow-up of 11.4 months, there has been one recurrence in both the laparoscopic purse-string groups and the laparoscopic external needle closure group, while none occurred in the Bassini herniorraphy group. This recurrence in the laparoscopic purse-string group occurred in a professional footballer, the second patient of the series, in whom only one purse-string had been applied. A video review of the initial laparoscopic repair and examination of the retrieved suture material, in this one case of recurrence, suggested that the suture material fractured probably as a result of trauma from the grasping forceps. The second recurrence in the laparoscopic external needle closure group occurred as a result of inappropriately spaced interrupted sutures. This enabled omental herniation between the sutures.

Discussion

In recent years there has been a rapid expansion in laparoscopic surgery and especially laparoscopic cholecystectomy [8]. Successful laparoscopic management of inguinal hernias has recently been reported in an experimental animal model by Ger and colleagues [9]. The rationale for such an approach is based on the observation that coincidental hernias found during the performance of an intra-abdominal procedure were effectively treated by closure of the internal hernial opening with stainless steel clips [5]. The present analysis demonstrates that indirect inguinal hernias may be managed safely, effectively and with minimal morbidity using a laparoscopic approach.

Laparoscopy affords excellent visualization of the vas deferens and inferior epigastric vessels allowing safe closure of the neck of the hernial sac. In a number of cases it was possible to invert the body of the sac into the peritoneal cavity and incorporate it into the purse-string suture thus completely obliterating the sac. The time required to perform the laparoscopic hernia repair will greatly improve with new technology. Of particular benefit will be the availability of a specifically designed clip applicator for the rapid closure of the neck of the sac [9]. Alternatively, extracorporeal suturing techniques may shorten operating time [7]. The laparoscopic repair may be reinforced by the use of a polypropylene (Marlex) mesh. This monofilament prosthetic material is non-allergenic, non-oncogenic and highly resistant to infection. It serves as an effective and permanent barrier to protrusion through the posterior wall of the inguinal canal and is readily incorporated into the tissues [10]. The Marlex patch can be expeditiously placed over the defect without tension or distortion of the surrounding tissues. Only a long-term follow-up will determine whether or not a Marlex patch should be used to avoid recurrence of the hernia.

A further advantage of the laparoscopic technique is the marked reduction of wound infection—up to 4.3% in patients who do not receive prophylactic antibiotics while undergoing standard herniorraphy [11]. As has been shown in the case of children, pneumoperitoneum is a safe and effective means of evaluating the contralateral groin for an occult hernia at the time of unilateral hernia repair [12]. Laparoscopic hernia repair allows simultaneous hernia repair with the advantages of only one admission, one anaesthetic, one operation and one period of convalescence. Following this technique, return to full activity is almost immediate and there are obvious economic advantages. Of particular interest is the low reading on the pain visual analogue scale obtained with this procedure 24 h postoperatively. Wound haematoma and groin pain can be greatly reduced with this procedure. Unfortunately, it is not possible to perform this procedure under local anaesthesia; however, this may well be a development in the future.

Finally, we would like to state that although we find our initial results encouraging, a cautious prospective trial will be necessary to thoroughly evaluate the laparoscopic techniques of hernia repair with or without Marlex patch placement with sufficient follow-up before this new technique can be freely recommended to patients.

References

1 Marcy HO. The cure of hernia. *JAMA* 1887; **8**: 589–592.
2 LaRoque GP. The intra-abdominal method of removing inguinal and femoral hernia. *Arch Surg* 1932; **24**: 189–203.
3 Andrews E. A method of herniotomy utilizing only white fascia. *Ann Surg* 1924; **80**: 225–238.
4 Vibits H, Pahle E. Recurrences after inguinal herniotomy in children. Long term follow-up. *Ann Chir Gynaecol* 1992; **81**: 300–302.
5 Ger R. The management of certain abdominal herniae by intra-abdominal closure of the neck of the sac. *Ann R Coll Surg Engl* 1982; **64**: 342–344.
6 Geraghty JG, Grace PA, Qureshi A, Bouchier-Hayes D, Osborne H. Simple new technique for laparoscopic hernia repair. *Br J Surg* 1994; **81**: 93.
7 Grace PA, Bouchier-Hayes D. A laparoscopic knot. *Br J Surg* 1992; **79**: 512.
8 Cuschieri A, Dubois F, Mouiel J, Mouret P, Becker H, Buess G, Trede M, Troidl H. The European experience with laparoscopic cholecystectomy. *Am J Surg* 1991; **161**: 385–387.
9 Ger R, Monroe K, Duvivier R, Mishrick A. Management of indirect inguinal hernias by laparoscopic closure of the neck of the sac. *Am J Surg* 1990; **159**: 370–373.
10 Lichtenstein IL, Schulman AG, Amid PK. Use of mesh to prevent recurrence of hernias. *Postgrad Med* 1990; **87**: 155–160.
11 Lazorthes F, Chiotasso P, Massip P, Materre JP, Sarkissian M. Local antibiotic prophylaxis in inguinal hernia repair. *Surg Gynaecol Obstet* 1992; **175**: 569–570.
12 Harrison CB, Kaplan GW, Scherz HC, Packer MG. Diagnostic pneumoperitoneum for the detection of clinically occult contralateral hernia in children. *J Urol* 1990; **144**: 510–511.

Chapter 13
Learning curve and training in laparoscopic hernia repair

C. Nduka and A. Darzi

Few technological advances in medicine have evolved as rapidly and engendered so much interest and debate as laparoscopic surgery. The proven advantages of laparoscopic cholecystectomy in terms of hospital stay, postoperative pain, cosmetic results and financial savings [1–7] have put considerable pressure on the surgical community to learn these new techniques promptly. The speed with which these techniques are being adopted has meant that guidelines on credentialling have fallen behind. Furthermore, reports of serious complications and even deaths have suggested that the training and evaluation of laparoscopic general surgeons needs urgent attention [8–15].

Laparoscopic surgical procedures involve skills that are unfamiliar to most general surgeons. Besides the manual dexterity and hand–eye coordination required of open surgery, performance of safe laparoscopic herniorrhaphy demands exceptional hand–instrument–monitor–eye coordination. The surgeon has to acquire the ability to operate through multiple punctures using an ever-increasing array of advanced equipment to achieve incision, dissection, haemostasis, stapling and suturing. Depth perception and tactile feedback are all but lost, as is the ability to perform complex manipulations.

The additional skills required of aspiring laparoscopic surgeons obviously do not come naturally. Even the simplest surgical procedures such as suturing and knot-tying need to be relearned. Furthermore, the surgical approach to inguinal hernia repair is completely different from that of the traditional repair. Unless the surgeon has an intimate knowledge of the endoscopically viewed anatomy of the inguinal region, there will always be a great potential for serious complications. Surgeons thus face the twin challenge of incorporating new techniques into the repertoire of experienced surgeons and of training junior surgeons *de novo*. Many laparoscopy courses are available in both Europe and the United States of America. However, concern has been expressed that some of these have been hurriedly and incompletely organized, allowing inadequately trained surgeons to practise unsupervised [10, 16, 17]. There has also been concern about the need to practise laparoscopic techniques on live animals [10], although this does not directly apply to the teaching of hernia repair.

Regarding the issue of training there are three important questions that need to be addressed. The first and most important is, 'what is the best method of teaching laparoscopic technique?'. Related to this is the question of whether this can be achieved in the context of a short course. The third and most neglected question is whether laparoscopic surgical skills can be reliably assessed. To address these issues of teaching, laparoscopic hernia surgery needs to be incorporated into the wider context of surgical training in general.

Surgeons have traditionally learned surgical skills by a process of supervised exposure and gradual operative experience [18, 19]. However, relatively little emphasis has been placed on the importance of teaching (and even less on evaluating) surgical skills [19–22]. Because the development of motor skills is an active learning process, surgical training ideally should be based on principles of learning theory [19]. Kopta has related learning theory to the acquisition of operative skills in orthopaedic surgery [20, 23]. He identified four determinants of surgical skill: speed, accuracy, economy of effort and adaptability [20]. One fundamental principle of motor skill development is that skill retention correlates with the level of initial proficiency, and not with practice, the type of training, or prior ability [24]. A second important principle is the need to minimize exposure to indiscriminate practice [23]. Such practice inevitably leads to the acquisition of faulty technique which is subsequently difficult to eradicate. These two principles have important implications for those teaching and learning laparoscopic surgery.

The fact that skill retention correlates with initial proficiency suggests that some general surgeons may not have the necessary hand–instrument–monitor–eye coordination to safely and efficiently perform laparoscopic procedures. Support for the suggestion that 'you either have it or you don't' may be derived from studies of a form of visual–spatial ability (field articulation) [25], and by personal observation of trainee laparoscopic surgeons. Unfortunately, there are no reliable predictors of technical skills that allow early identification of those possessing (or lacking) the desired psychomotor attributes [22]. Indeed the basic question of inherent skill and aptitude levels may be equally applied to the learning and performance of traditional open surgery. A second implication of learning theory relates to the provision of adequate feedback, both from the trainee surgeon and from more experienced surgeons. The importance of continual feedback cannot be overemphasized as deficiencies in training are unlikely to be corrected without mechanisms for reliable and systematic feedback [20]. Nicks *et al.* have evaluated the relative role of cognitive instruction, autonomous practice, and supervised practice in the performance of simple surgical tasks in medical students [26]. They found that supervised practice resulted in optimal development of technical skills. Furthermore, they argued that supervised instruction was important before the students encountered practice opportunities in the operating room. This supports the provision of psychomotor skills laboratories or craft workshops [18, 19, 27] as used in many training centres (Fig. 13.1).

There are no realistic animal models of inguinal hernia. However, using animals to gain general laparoscopic surgical skills is an important issue that has moral, philosophical, legal and financial implications [28]. As this practice is illegal in the UK, many aspiring laparoscopic surgeons go abroad to gain what they feel is an important part of their training. The importance of practice in live anaesthetized animals (usually pigs) has been stressed by several authors [10, 11, 29–32]. Indeed, neither the Society of American Gastrointestinal Endoscopic Surgeons (SAGES) nor the American Society for Surgery of the Alimentary Tract (SSAT) [9] allow general

Figure 13.1

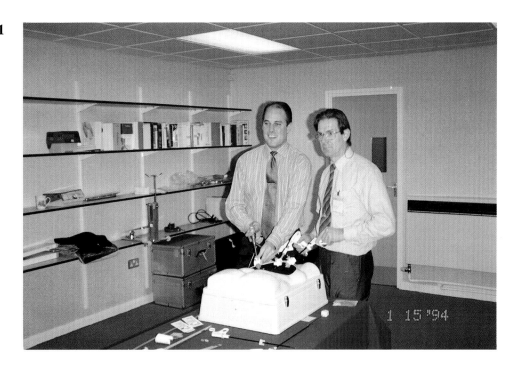

surgeons to practise laparoscopy without prior practice on animals. Indeed one author goes as far as stating that a didactic course alone, without the opportunity for experience with live animals, constitutes inadequate training [10]. However, gynaecologists have long discovered that sufficient *supervised* practice is a safe and equivalent substitute for animal simulation. The high cost of maintaining and disposing of animal training models adds weight to this argument.

Determining the ideal number of supervised procedures necessary for a surgeon to be allowed to operate unsupervised is difficult without a reliable method of assessing a surgeon's competence. There are five main methods of assessing technical skills [33]:

1 recording a log of procedures performed;
2 the use of direct observation;
3 direct observation with structured objective criteria;
4 the use of simulator models with criteria;
5 videorecording procedures.

Recording a log of procedures performed is relatively easy but lacks validity because it does not account for whether the procedure was performed adequately. The use of direct observation with structured objective criteria is a useful, if time-consuming, mode of assessment. Such a method has been used to evaluate junior orthopaedic surgeons and has been shown to be both reliable and valid [20]. Animal (e.g. pig) or artificial simulators, if used in conjunction with structured criteria, are also highly reliable. The validity of this method is proportional to the realism of the simulator [33]. For example, many surgeons practise laparoscopic dissection by peeling a grape placed in a simulator. While the skills gained from such an exercise are undoubtedly useful, success in performing the task only correlates with true proficiency in as much as a grape correlates with human anatomy. Assessment of skills should therefore ideally take place *in vivo*.

Videorecording of procedures is a highly valid and reliable method of assessment [23, 34]. It has been suggested that this method has a major disadvantage of being costly [22]. However, this is not the case with laparoscopic surgery: the necessary equipment (camera, videorecorder and monitor) is already present. Furthermore, the new generation of laparoscopic surgical simulators incorporate standard camcorders, providing trainee surgeons with an inexpensive means of practising basic techniques. The means for personal and supervised practice of laparoscopic techniques are thus already in place. A surgeon's performance over time can be monitored by compiling a library of procedures performed—a type of surgical video-diary. An interesting step would be the formulation of a structured objective evaluation system for laparoscopic surgery, similar to the one formulated by Kopta for orthopaedic surgeons [20]. Another advantage of having videotaped laparoscopic procedures is that they allow novice surgeons to be shown repeatedly the correct method of performing a given procedure. Educational objectives can therefore be clearly defined and exposure to faulty techniques minimized. Video demonstrations are extensively used on our course and each participant receives a delegate pack containing literature and a video explaining the operative technique.

We recently conducted a poll of 20 surgeons in order to gauge what they felt should be the minimum training requirements for an aspiring laparoscopic surgeon. All were experienced in laparoscopy (had performed over 50 laparoscopic cholecystectomies) and had previously attended a laparoscopic herniorrhaphy training course (Table 13.1). The general consensus was that the attendance of a recognized course together with on-the-job training with an experienced surgeon should be mandatory before unsupervised practice is permitted (Fig. 13.2). The recent establishment of Minimally Invasive Therapy Training Units by the Royal College of Surgeons in England may go some way to satisfying the need for expert training. The issue of reliable surgical skills still needs to be addressed.

Figure 13.2

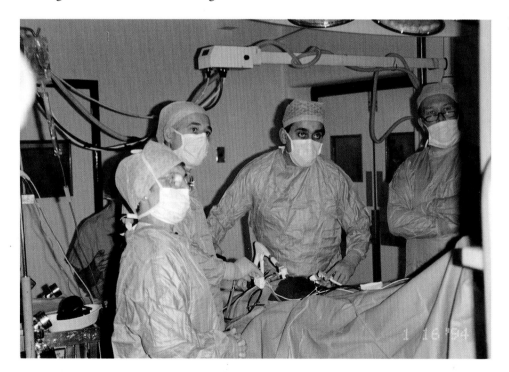

Table 13.1
Suggested ideal training requirements before unsupervised practice.

Ideal training requirement	Positive responses
On-the-job training with experienced surgeon	20 (100%)
Attendance of recognized course	20 (100%)
Written examination (e.g. endoscopic anatomy)	4 (20%)
Specified no. of assisted procedures*	12 (60%)
Formal certification by experienced surgeon	8 (40%)
Probationary period and audit of morbidity†	10 (50%)

*Mean no. of assisted procedures suggested = 6.7 (range 5–10).
†Mean no. of cases suggested for audit = 16.5 (range 5–20).

An exciting advance in computer technology, known as virtual reality, promises to revolutionize the field of surgical training [35, 36]. Laparoscopic surgical simulators are under development which display a 'virtual' representation of the abdominal cavity on a video monitor. Any movements made by the operator are represented on the screen. Intra-abdominal organs such as the gallbladder can be grasped and resected. It is hoped that in the near future virtual reality surgical simulators will be able to mimic real operations—right down to bleeding blood vessels. Apart from eliminating the unnecessary slaughter of animals, such a system will have the potential advantage of being able to accurately mimic diseased organs or abnormal anatomy, and to provide a means of objective assessment.

References

1 Spaw A, Reddick E, Olsen D. Laparoscopic laser cholecystectomy: Analysis of 500 procedures. *Surg Laparosc Endosc* 1991; **1**: 2–7.
2 The Southern Surgeons Club. A prospective analysis of 1518 laparoscopic cholecystectomies. *N Engl J Med* 1991; **324**: 1073–1078.
3 Graves HA Jr, Ballinger JF, Anderson WJ. Appraisal of laparoscopic cholecystectomy. *Ann Surg* 1991; **213**: 655–664.
4 Schirmer BD, Edge SB, Dix J *et al.* Laparoscopic cholecystectomy. *Ann Surg* 1991; **213**: 665–667.
5 Peters JH, Ellison EC, Innes JT *et al.* Safety and efficacy of laparoscopic cholecystectomy. *Ann Surg* 1991; **213**: 3–12.
6 Grace PA, Quereshi A, Coleman J, Keane R, McEntee G, Broe P, Osborne H, Bouchier-Hayes D. Reduced postoperative hospitalisation after laparoscopic cholecystectomy. *Br J Surg* 1991; **78**: 160–162.
7 Dubois F, Icard P, Berthelot G, Levard H. Coelioscopic cholecystectomy. *Ann Surg* 1990; **211**: 60–63.
8 Private hospitals ban laparoscopic surgery [news]. *Br Med J* 1993; **306**: 1227.
9 Tompkins RK. Laparoscopic cholecystectomy: threat or opportunity? *Arch Surg* 1990; **125**: 1245.
10 Dent TL. Training, credentialling and granting of clinical privileges for laparoscopic general surgery. *Am J Surg* 1991; **161**: 399–403.
11 Asbun HJ, Reddick EJ. Credentialling in laparoscopic surgery: A survey of physicians. *J Laparoendosc Surg* 1992; **2**: 27–32.
12 Wickham JEA. Minimally invasive therapy (Editorial) *Minimally Invasive Therapy* 1993; **2**: 45.
13 Corbitt JD Jr. Laparoscopic herniorrhaphy. *Surg Laparosc Endosc* 1991; **1**: 23–25.
14 Dion Y-M, Morin J. Laparoscopic inguinal herniorrhaphy. *Can J Surg* 1992; **35**: 209–212.
15 Ger R, Mishrick A, Hurwitz J, Romero C, Oddsen R. Management of groin hernias by laparoscopy. *World J Surg* 1993; **17**: 46–50.
16 Kirwan WO, Kaar TK, Waldron R. Starting laparoscopic cholecystectomy—The pig as a training model. *Irish J Med Sci* 1991; **160**: 243–246.
17 Cuschieri A. The laparoscopic revolution—walk carefully before we run. *J R Coll Surg Edinb* 1989; **34**: 295.

18 Bevan PG, Craft workshops in surgery. *Br J Surg* 1986; **73**: 1–2.

19 Barnes RW. Surgical handicraft: teaching and learning surgical skills. *Am J Surg* 1987; **153**: 422–427.

20 Kopta JA. An approach to the evaluation of operative skills. *Surgery* 1971; **70**: 297–303.

21 Spencer FC. Observations on the teaching of operative technique. *Am Coll Surg* 1983; **68**: 3–6.

22 Reznick RK. Teaching and testing technical skills. *Am J Surg* 1993; **165**: 358–361.

23 Kopta JA. The development of motor skills in orthopedic education. *Clin Orthop* 1971; **75**: 80–85.

24 Fleishman EA, Parker JF Jr. Factors in the retention and relearning of perceptual-motor skill. *J Exp Psychol* 1962; **64**: 215–226.

25 Gibbons RD, Baker RJ, Skinner DB. Field articulation testing: A predictor of technical skills in surgical residents. *J Surg Res* 1986; **41**: 53–57.

26 Nicks CM, Nelson CL, Lang NP. Use of the surgical skills laboratory for teaching medical students. *Focus Surg Ed* 1986; **3**: 13.

27 Lippert FG III, Farmer JA. *Psychomotor Skills in Orthopedic Surgery*. Williams & Wilkins, Baltimore, 1984.

28 Cooper AJ, Johnson CD. Animal experimentation. *Br J Surg* 1991; **78**: 1409–1411.

29 Bailey RW, Imbembo AL, Zucker KA. Establishment of a laparoscopic cholecystectomy training program. *Am Surg* 1991; **57**: 231–236.

30 Cohen MM. Initial experience with laparoscopic cholecystectomy in a teaching hospital. *Can J Surg* 1992; **35**: 59–63.

31 Cuschieri A, Berci G, McSherry CK. Laparoscopic cholecystectomy. *Am J Surg* 1990; **159**: 273.

32 Zucker KA, Bailey RW, Graham SM, Scovil W, Imbembo AL. Training for laparoscopy. *World J Surg* 1993; **17**: 2–7.

33 Watts J, Feldman WB. Assessment of technical skills. In: Neufeld VR, Norman GR (eds). *Assessing Clinical Competence*. Springer, New York, 1985: 259–274.

34 Lui P, Miller E, Herg G. Videotape reliability: a method of evaluation of a clinical performance examination. *J Med Educ* 1980; **55**: 713–715.

35 Satava RM. Robotics, telepresence and virtual reality: a critical analysis of the future of surgery. *Min Inv Surg* 1992; **1**: 357–363.

36 Satava RM. Virtual reality surgical simulator: the first steps. *Surg Endosc* 1993; **7**: 203–205.

Further reading

Andrew BJ. The use of behavioural checklists to assess physical exam skills. *J Med Educ* 1977; **52**: 589–590.

Cuschieri A, Shimi S, Nathanson LK. Laparoscopic reduction, crural repair and fundoplication of large hiatal hernia. *Am J Surg* 1992; **163**: 425–430.

Darzi A, Hill ADK, Henry MM, Guillou PJ, Monson JRT. Laparoscopic assisted surgery of the colon. Operative technique. *Endosc Surg* 1993; **1**: 13–15.

Delaitre B, Maignien B, Icard P. Laparoscopic splenectomy. *Br J Surg* 1992; **79**: 1334.

Delaney PV, Quill RD, Kalizser M. Assessment of operative surgical skills. *J Ir Med Assoc* 1978; **71**: 13.

Fiel NJ, Griffin PE, McNeil JA *et al*. A model for evaluating student clinical psychomotor skills. *J Med Educ* 1979; **54**: 511–513.

Harden RM, Stephenson M, Downie W. Assessment of clinical competence using an objective structured examination. *Br Med J* 1975; **i**: 447–451.

Kathkouda N, Mouiel J. A new technique of surgical treatment of chronic duodenal ulcer without laparotomy by videocelioscopy. *Am J Surg* 1991; **161**: 361–364.

Mouret P, Francois Y, Vignal J *et al*. Laparoscopic treatment of perforated peptic ulcer. *Br J Surg* 1990; **77**: 1006.

Oakes DD, Sherck JP, Brodsky JB *et al*. Therapeutic thoracoscopy. *J Thorac Cardiovasc Surg* 1984; **87**: 269–273.

Paget GW. Laparoscopic repair of inguinal hernia. *Med J Aust* 1992; **156**: 508–510.

Paterson-Brown S, Garden OJ, Carter DC. Laparoscopic cholecystectomy. *Br J Surg* 1991; **78**: 1431–1432.

Sclinkert RT. Laparoscopic assisted right hemicolectomy. *Dis Colon Rectum* 1991; **34**: 1030–1031.

Society of American Gastrointestinal Endoscopic Surgeons. Granting of privileges for laparoscopic general surgery. *Am J Surg* 1991; **161**: 324–325.

Soper NJ, Stockmann PT, Dunnegan DL, Ashley SW. Laparoscopic cholecystectomy. The new 'gold standard'? *Arch Surg* 1992; **127**: 917–921.

Wastell C. Laparoscopic cholecystectomy. Better for patients and the health service (Editorial). *Br Med J* 1991; **302**: 304–305.

Chapter 14
Principles and complications of diathermy in endoscopic surgery

C. Nduka, J.R.T. Monson and A. Darzi

Electrosurgical devices play a vital role in the ever-expanding number of laparoscopic procedures, from gynaecology, through general surgery to urology. The minimal access nature of laparoscopic surgery makes the correct use of diathermy particularly important for the safe performance of a procedure. This is especially the case with laparoscopic hernia repair, which requires an unfamiliar surgical approach and involves the use of electrical energy in close proximity to a number of important structures. All surgeons should be aware of the problems that may arise during an operation as such awareness allows potential complications to be avoided or effectively dealt with as they arise.

Electrosurgical principles

The field of neurosurgery was revolutionized by Harvey Cushing's publication, in 1928, of a series of 500 cranial procedures in which tumour removal and control of bleeding was facilitated by using an electrosurgical unit designed by W.T. Bovie [1]. The observed tissue effect was the result of a high-frequency current producing heat in and around an electrical arc generated by the so-called Bovie unit.

Surgical diathermy (electrocoagulation) relies on the principle that high-frequency current can be passed through the body with no effects other than the production of heat [2]. The amount of heat produced by the current is inversely proportional to the electrode area. Two types of diathermy electrode are commonly used: monopolar and bipolar. With a monopolar diathermy probe, one electrode (return electrode or ground plate) is large (e.g. 100 cm^2) and the other is small (<1 cm^2). This small or 'active' electrode is used to control the current density, i.e. the current per unit area. The rate of heat production and resulting therapeutic effect is a direct function of the current density and depends on: (i) the applied voltage; (ii) the area of active electrode in contact with the tissue; and (iii) the tissue resistance. Current enters the patient via the active electrode and exits from the return electrode site. The latter should have a large surface area to protect against high current density and therefore skin burns. It is important to note that, with monopolar diathermy, current can pass from the active to the return electrode via any route (single probe or forceps). In contrast, bipolar diathermy employs current flow only between the two sides of the forceps, with a localization of the tissue effect.

As Bovie and Cushing discovered, a continuous high-frequency current produces a cutting effect, whereas an intermittent high-frequency current causes coagulation of vessels with little or no cutting. Haemostasis alone is accomplished when the waveform is pulsed (or damped) on and off, with on times being one-fifth to one-tenth as long as off times [3]. A modified or blended effect of cutting and coagulation is produced by longer on/off time ratios, shown in Fig. 14.1.

In a unipolar electrode, electrical energy is relatively quickly diffused in tissue. Specifically, a unipolar electrode's current density falls off as the square of the radius of a circle from the point source. With the bipolar electrode, current density is largely concentrated at the tip because tissue contact completes a circuit between two wires only 3 mm apart (Fig. 14.2). This density falls off as the fourth power of the distance from the electrode, suggesting that tissue thermal energy can be more precisely localized, thus preserving deeper submucosal and muscular layers intact [4]. As a consequence, bipolar electrodes function at a much lower power output than monopolar ones [5]. They are also more effective in saline solution than in water, as water has a high resistance. Conversely, the monopolar electrode works poorly in saline owing to the low-resistance saline presenting the current with alternative paths and carrying much of the current away from the tissue directly under the electrode.

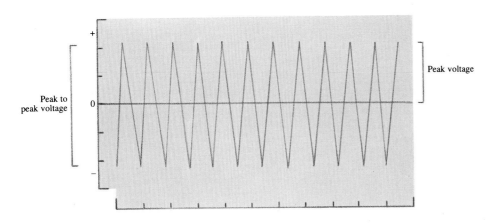

Figure 14.1
(a) Pure or cutting waveform.
(b) Damped coagulating waveform.

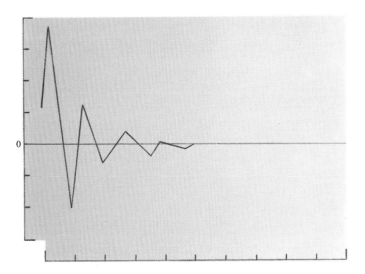

Figure 14.2
Current densities with monopolar (right) and bipolar electrodes (left). With the monopolar electrode, current density is proportional to r^2; with the bipolar electrode it is proportional to r^4, thus concentrating the electrical energy at the electrode tip.

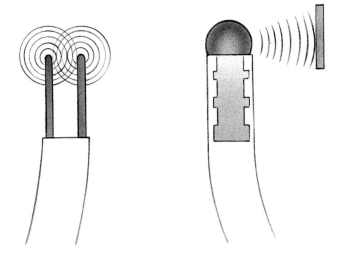

Monopolar or bipolar diathermy?

The main advantage of monopolar over bipolar diathermy is its ease of use [6]. Monopolar methods have also been shown to be more effective at achieving haemostasis in animal models of bleeding gastric ulcers [6]. This is related to the differences in fall-off of current densities and the anatomy of the bleeding ulcer. Because of its deeper penetration, monopolar electrocoagulation tends to coagulate vessels deep in the submucosa, or in the muscular area, as they branch upward towards the ulcer base [7]. The greater penetration of current density with monopolar techniques is an advantage for haemostasis, but is also one of the major causes of complications associated with its use. The most frequent serious complications reported are thermal injuries to the bowel.

The major advantage of bipolar diathermy is the reduction in tissue damage. Several studies have reported satisfactory haemostasis with less tissue injury than monopolar techniques [4, 8, 9]. Because each jaw has the same surface area, the electrons only heat the tissue interposed between. This process is self-limiting; as soon as the cells are charred and completely dehydrated, the current ceases to pass, thus avoiding damage to the surrounding tissues [10]. In a comparison of various coagulation techniques, Riedel and co-workers demonstrated that monopolar techniques produce an area of coagulation twice that of a bipolar electrode, and more than four times that of the carbon dioxide laser [11].

Irreversible tissue damage due to protein denaturation occurs in the temperature range of 55–60°C [12]. Ramsay and co-workers compared the intraluminal tissue heat from both types of electrode applied to rabbit bladders. They found an average rise of 19.9°C above core temperature in the lumen adjacent to the monopolar electrode, which was probably sufficient to cause protein denaturation. In contrast, the bipolar technique only produced a maximum temperature rise of 3.5°C under similar circumstances [13]. Figure 14.3 shows the conduction of heat measured intraluminally from a site of diathermy application.

Monopolar diathermy therefore causes deeper damage due to the current traversing the tissue to the ground plate. Interestingly, the diameter of injury with either technique may be more closely related to the electrode diameter than to the

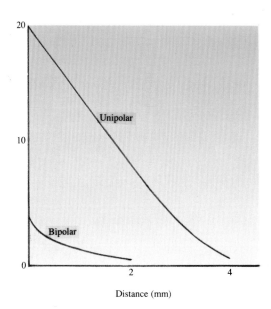

Figure 14.3
Conduction of heat from the point of diathermy.

absolute current passed [5]. As with monopolar diathermy, the tissue necrosis resulting from bipolar techniques varies directly with the duration, energy, and force of electrode application [8].

Most of the advantages of bipolar over monopolar diathermy are due to the elimination of the ground plate. Monopolar diathermy requires that the whole patient should behave as an electrolyte solution, whereas with bipolar diathermy the production of heat does not depend on electrical conduction between active and return electrodes. As a consequence: (i) there is no electrical interference with the function of implanted electrical devices [13]; (ii) bipolar diathermy operates at lower currents thereby reducing nerve and muscle stimulation [5]; (iii) there is no possibility of sparking [10]; (iv) bipolar electrodes can operate in normal saline bathing solutions [14]; and (v) there is no capacitance effect, possibly due to a cancelling out of the waveform [3]. There is also a reduction in the production of smoke [11], a factor that may be important in accidental bowel injury. The main criticism of bipolar diathermy is that it is more difficult to use [6]. This is a primary reason for employing monopolar diathermy in preference to bipolar techniques. Another reason is that the low energy output of bipolar systems may be insufficient to coagulate larger blood vessels [3]. A further drawback is the adherence of coagulated tissue to the bipolar forceps [6, 11], which may require repeated cleaning. However, the possibility of accidental bowel injuries occurring with bipolar diathermy is minimal. This would require the inadvertent grasping of tissue together with current application. Even if this was to occur, it is very unlikely to pass unnoticed so measures could be taken to limit the extent of injury.

Aetiology of accidental diathermy injuries

Most of the large series reporting the incidence of electrosurgical burns to the bowel come from gynaecological procedures performed in the 1970s [15–17]. The overall incidence of thermal injury associated with laparoscopy has been reported at between one and two patients per 1000 operated upon [18]. Peterson and co-workers [19] have reported two deaths resulting from thermal bowel injury following the use of unipolar devices.

As in the cases reported above, electrical injuries to the bowel are usually unrecognized at the time of occurrence [17]. Patients with unrecognized bowel injuries generally present 3–7 days after injury with complaints of fever and abdominal pain. However, reported intervals from time of occurrence of injury to onset of symptoms vary from 18 h to 14 days [17]. At laparotomy or laparoscopy, the gross appearance of both traumatic and electrical injuries is the same: the perforation is usually surrounded by a white area of necrosis. Microscopic examination of thermal injuries shows the persistence of necrotic tissue without a leucocytic infiltrate. In contrast, puncture injuries exhibit a rapid capillary proliferation, polymorphonuclear infiltration, and fibrin deposition at the injury site [20]. Since most bowel injuries with monopolar devices are unrecognized at the time of operation, the reasons for their occurrence can only be speculated on. The commonest explanations for thermal injuries occurring during laparoscopy are as follows (Fig. 14.4):

Figure 14.4

(a) Direct coupling between an activated electrode and a metal instrument, out of view of the laparoscope. (b) Electrical isolation of the fallopian tube following coagulation may cause the current to return to the ground plate via the bowel, causing a burn. (c) Electrical isolation of the gallbladder and cystic duct may cause a burn by the same mechanism. (d) Capacitance induced in a metal cannula may cause a burn if the current cannot dissipate via the abdominal wall.

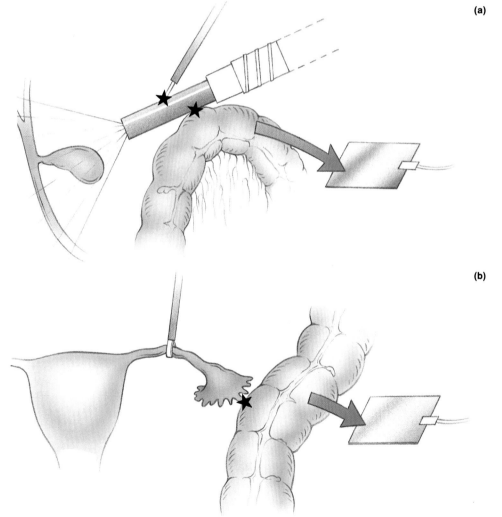

(a)

(b)

Figure 14.4(c), (d)

(c)

(d)

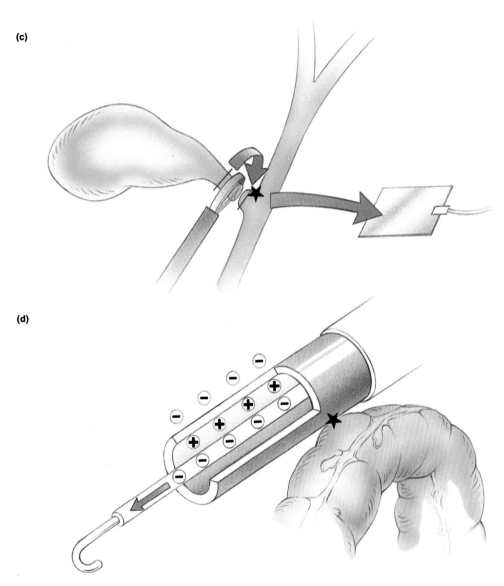

1 Inadvertent touching or grasping of the bowel during the application of current.
2 Direct coupling (or unintended contact) between a portion of bowel and a metal instrument, which is touching the activated probe (or connected to it by an electrical arc).
3 Insulation breaks in the electrodes.
4 Direct sparking to bowel from the diathermy probe.
5 In laparoscopic sterilization, current passing along the fallopian tube and jumping from the fimbriated end to the bowel.

The first theory probably explains the majority of thermal injuries. Indeed, several studies have noted the difficulty in controlling the extent of tissue injury—even when application of the probe is under strict control. Piercey and co-workers [21] found that, despite the addition of an analogue computer to control energy delivery, deep tissue injury occurred in an unpredictable manner; the computer did not decrease tissue injury. The pressure of electrode application has a marked influence on the depth of injury. A theoretical factor that may also be important is the current pathway. Current passes randomly from the active electrode to the ground plate, following the pathway of least impedance [21]. If the pathway is narrow, current density is high resulting in more coagulation and/or necrosis than expected. Differential tissue cooling due to variable vasculature or the time elapsed between electrode applications may also play a part in determining the extent of injury [21].

There had been controversy about the possibility of bowel burns being the result of contact with hot, recently cauterized tissue or with a recently activated electrode. DiGiovanni and co-workers have investigated this possibility in rabbits, but were unable to produce any histological evidence of bowel injury [22]. Contact between the activated diathermy probe and the metal trocar sleeve (or other conductive instruments) is unlikely to result in a bowel burn. This is because the relatively large area of trocar in electrical contact with the abdominal wall (about 3–4 cm^2 with a 12 mm trocar) would provide an alternative low-resistance pathway for current dissipation. However, *in vitro* studies have shown that insulated cannulae which prevent the dissipation of current may cause bowel burns.

Direct sparking from the monopolar probe to the bowel has been suggested by several authors [3, 10, 15]. In fact a 15 000 V pressure can push electrons more than 1 cm in air under certain atmospheric conditions [3]. As currents used to coagulate the fallopian tubes must course through the patient's body to reach the ground plate, electrical sparking is a potential threat, especially with the older high-voltage electrosurgical units. The past use of such units in tubal cauterization has been blamed for a proportion of these accidental burns [15]. Fortunately modern low-voltage high-frequency units operate with a maximum peak voltage of 300–600 V so sparking by this mechanism is unlikely. However, repeated use of instruments often leads to insulation failure as a result of wear and tear. Although not always visible, defects in insulation may lead to direct delivery of almost all of the electrical energy beyond the view of the operator [23]. Under these circumstances, large currents are not necessary to produce a full-thickness injury.

Soderstrom proposed an explanation for bowel injuries that invokes the property of capacitance. A capacitor exists wherever an insulating material separates two conductors that have a potential difference between them. When an active electrode is passed through a (non-conducting) fibreglass trocar, the result is a tube within a tube across which a difference in electrical potential exists. When current passes through the active electrode, the laparoscope itself becomes a capacitor (see Fig. 14.4d). Measurements have shown that from 50 to 70% of the active electrode current is induced into the laparoscope wall [3]. Thus when the metal part of the laparoscope comes into contact with the bowel, a pin-point burn results as the electrons find a return pathway. A recent study [23] has shown that such capacitive coupling may occur *in vivo* and result in a full-thickness injury. Such burns are more likely to occur when small trocars are used. This situation does not arise with all-metal trocars as the area in electrical contact with the abdominal wall is sufficient for the non-thermal dissipation of current.

An intriguing possibility is that during laparoscopic tubal sterilization thermal injuries can result from the passage of current along the fallopian tube to the bowel (Fig. 14.3). When a fallopian tube is coagulated, the fimbral end becomes electrically isolated. Under these conditions it is possible that the bowel may represent the path of least electrical resistance to the ground plate, either by direct contact with the fibrium or by sparking. The small dimensions of a fibrium could thus result in a sufficiently high current density to cause a burn. It is not clear whether this mechanism actually plays a part in the creation of thermal injuries, but *in vitro* experiments may demonstrate its feasibility. If this mechanism is operating, one could postulate that such injuries could arise during other laparoscopic procedures that require prolonged high-current coagulation, such as appendicectomy and cholecystectomy.

Despite the many theories to explain thermal injuries with monopolar diathermy, there is one point of common agreement. Electrical energy under different conditions can behave in an uncontrolled and erratic manner that is often beyond our ability to predict.

Improving electrosurgical safety

The likelihood of accidental electrical burns may be reduced by attainment of a perfect visual image with an adequate pneumoperitoneum [17]. The view may be further improved by use of a 30° forward oblique telescope [24]. The latter is particularly helpful in procedures requiring that the instruments cross loops of bowel, such as appendicectomy and herniorrhaphy.

Excessive use of diathermy should be avoided because cleavage planes can be obscured by the heat-induced contraction of tissues. Before applying the electrode to vital structures, the intensity of the coagulation current should be tested to ensure the desired tissue effect. The use of an instrument with suction–irrigation capabilities is also suggested [25] because it allows the surgeon to keep the operative field much cleaner. Most importantly, diathermy should never be used blindly to control bleeding; the surgeon should be willing to convert to an open operation when the dissection becomes bloody or otherwise difficult [25].

It has been reported that approximately 43% of unprepared bowels contain a potentially explosive mixture of hydrogen, methane and oxygen [26]. Explosive injuries following activation of diathermy are thankfully rare, but have been fatal [27–29]. To prevent future occurrences, the bowel must be properly prepared in procedures exposing the diathermy to bowel gases. Furthermore, mannitol-containing bowel preparations which may promote methane production should be avoided.

In addition to the general points outlined above, there are a number of measures that can be taken specifically to improve the safety of monopolar techniques. Excessive thermal damage may be prevented by ensuring that a voltage of not more than 200 V (soft coagulation) is used. At this voltage, damage to the instrument tips (including scissors) is minimized, and electrical sparking is unlikely. Aside from excessive current application, the greatest contribution to accidental injuries probably arises from inappropriate or inadequate insulation. Inappropriate insulation is involved in the aetiology of both capacitance and direct coupling burns. If conductive trocars and anchoring devices are used, any 'stray current' can be safely dissipated via the abdominal wall (discussed above). This last point has been emphasized by several authors [30], and is recommended by the American Food and Drug Administration (FDA) [23]. Proper insulation of the electrode is also necessary and may be facilitated by the use of commercially available dynamically monitored shields. Safety may be further improved by the use of the insulated electrosurgical hook knife. This instrument allows tenting of vessels before the activation of current, thus limiting the spread of injury. A problem with this instrument is its tendency to become entangled in omentum or other tissues. It also requires repeated cleaning to ensure optimal efficiency.

Use of a ground plate in monopolar diathermy is mandatory. Metal ground plates must be covered with the appropriate conductive jelly to obtain optimal contact with the patient. In many newer models, the ground plate has a sensor that recognizes the resistance of human tissue [31]. If the resistance changes due to displacement of the ground plate, the generator automatically stops and sounds a warning.

Occasionally, two monopolar probes may be plunged into one generator, either because more than one instrument is repeatedly required during an operation (e.g. hook knife and coagulating forceps), or because of incompatibility between the instrument lead and the generator socket. It is important to note that, with this arrangement, both monopolar electrodes are activated when one of the probes is being used; the redundant probe is usually safely stored in a plastic sheath. Under these circumstances cutaneous electrosurgical burns may result from careless placing of the redundant probe. To prevent these injuries, the use of two monopolar probes should be avoided. If this is not practical, meticulous care must be taken to ensure that the redundant probe is not in direct or indirect contact with the skin (e.g. via spilt saline irrigation fluid).

Bipolar methods are safer and should be used in preference to monopolar electrodes, particularly in anatomically crowded situations. However, bipolar diathermy is very limited at performing dissection, a reason for many surgeons preferring monopolar techniques. It has been suggested that bipolar diathermy may be made even safer by using a microprocessor-controlled generator [32]. When applied to a vessel, this device automatically initiates and ends coagulation when optimal vessel occlusion has been achieved. Proper evaluation of the additional benefits of this method has yet to be reported.

Diathermy injuries during laparoscopic hernia repair

During laparoscopic herniorrhaphy, diathermy is commonly used for dividing the peritoneum. Problems may arise if the patient is not sufficiently tilted in the Trendelenburg position causing the bowel to lie too close to the inguinal region. The operative field is thus obscured with the result that the bowel is susceptible to accidental burns by the mechanisms described above. Diathermy injuries are most likely to occur at the level of the rectosigmoid or caecum in a left- or right-sided hernia repair, respectively. If noticed, superficial injuries may be treated proactively with a laparoscopic purse-string suture placed beyond the margins of the thermally affected tissue. The urinary bladder and the ureters are also at risk. In particular, excessive diathermy should not be used when dividing the median umbilical ligament as high levels of thermal energy may be transmitted directly to the bladder. This is especially so with monopolar diathermy (see Fig. 14.3).

Alternatives to diathermy

Lasers

There has been much debate concerning the relative advantages of lasers over conventional diathermy [24]. There are three commonly used lasers, each having specific wavelengths: the Nd-YAG laser (infrared); the KTP laser (green light); and the argon laser (blue light). The ability of laser energy to heat tissue is dependent on power density (analogous to current density), the laser wavelength, and the tissue pigmentation. A major disadvantage of laser energy is that it is highly absorbed by dark pigments. Thus, in a large or briskly bleeding vessel, the coagulated superficial layers tend to inhibit further penetration of energy. As a consequence, when charring occurs over a bleeding vessel, the only hope of further photocoagulation is to remove the blackened superficial layer [24]. In contrast, diathermy is unaffected by the colour of tissues to be coagulated (although current spread will be limited by extreme tissue desiccation).

Unfortunately there are no prospective data comparing the performance of lasers and diathermy. However, two retrospective studies have found diathermy faster, cheaper and better at haemostasis [24] in laparoscopic cholecystectomy. This view is held by several authors [24, 35, 42, 43]. The high cost, technical requirements, additional staff and size of laser devices further contribute to their lack of appeal.

Ultrasonic devices

Ultrasonic scalpels are based on the principle that voltage applied across a piezoelectric crystal creates a mechanical stress. The cavtron ultrasonic surgical aspirator (CUSA) consists of a pencil-grip surgical handpiece containing a transducer that oscillates a titanium tip longitudinally at 23 kHz. The vibration is imperceptible, but sufficient heat is generated for dissection. These devices have the major advantage of allowing selective tissue fragmentation. Collagen-rich structures such as blood vessels and ureters are left intact [44], so that they can be secured before division. Ultrasonic dissection has been used in open general surgery for liver resection [45]. In laparoscopy, these devices have been used to aid colonic mobilization, for separation of the gallbladder from the liver (particularly when the organ is shrunken, fibrotic or intrahepatic), and for dissection of the common duct during laparoscopic supraduodenal exploration [46, 47].

The harmonic scalpel works on the same principle as the CUSA, except that the vibration frequency of the tip is much higher, in the harmonic range. The result is a cutting rather than a plane separating effect, with sufficient heat produced by friction to gently coagulate the cut surfaces. The potential advantages of ultrasonic devices over electrosurgical techniques have yet to be evaluated.

Conclusion

Bipolar electrodes are safer yet have a limited ability to perform dissection; monopolar techniques are easier but should not be used in anatomically crowded regions, or near delicate structures. Innovations in diathermy design may improve safety but have not been fully evaluated. Because advanced laparoscopic procedures such as herniorrhaphy and colon resection often require that instruments cross loops of bowel, the risk of thermal injuries may be considerably increased. Consequently, the importance of adequate visualization and use of bipolar diathermy, where possible, cannot be overemphasized. The limited number of large series of laparoscopic hernia repairs means that it is not yet possible to comment on the incidence of thermal injury. Present alternatives to electrosurgical methods (lasers and ultrasonic devices) may be of some additional benefit in the future. These benefits will need to be weighed up against the additional cost of the new technologies. However, it is important to stress that, with regard to the safety of any potentially hazardous technique, there is no real substitute for adequate training and supervision.

References

1 Cushing H. Electrosurgery as an aid to the removal of intracranial tumours. *Surg Gynaecol Obstet* 1928; **47**: 751–784.
2 Kopchok GE, White RA. Hemostatic and dissecting devices: Safety considerations and comparison of various modalities. In: White RA, Klein SR (eds) *Endoscopic Surgery*. Mosby Year Book, St. Louis, 1991: 61–73.
3 Soderstrom RM. Electrical safety in laparoscopy. In: Phillips JM (ed.) *Endoscopy in Gynaecology*. Downey, California, 1978: 306–311.
4 Moore JP, Silvis SE, Vennes JA. Evaluation of bipolar electrocoagulation in canine stomachs. *Gastro Endosc* 1978; **24**: 148–151.
5 Tucker RD, Kramulowsky EV, Bedell E, Platz C. A comparison of urologic application of bipolar versus monopolar: Five French electrosurgical probes. *J Urol* 1989; **141**: 662–665.
6 Johnston JH, Jensen DM, Mautner W. Comparison of endoscopic electrocoagulation and laser photocoagulation of bleeding canine gastric ulcers. *Gastroenterology* 1982; **82**: 904–910.
7 Papp JP. State of the art: Endoscopic electrocoagulation of actively bleeding arterial upper gastrointestinal lesions. *Am J Gastroenterol* 1979; **71**: 516–521.
8 Protell RL, Gilbert D, Silverstein F. Computer-assisted electrocoagulation: bipolar vs monopolar in the treatment of experimental canine gastric ulcer bleeding. *Gastroenterology* 1981; **80**: 451–455.
9 Veerhoeven AGM *et al*. A new multipolar coagulation electrode for endoscopic haemostasis. In: Van Maercke YFM, Van Moer EMJ (eds) *Stomach Diseases. Current Status*. Excerpta Medica, Amsterdam, 1981: 216–221.
10 Rioux JE, Cloutier D. A new bipolar instrument for laparoscopic tubal sterilization. *Am J Obstet Gynecol* 1974; **119**: 737.
11 Riedel HH, Corts-Kleinwort G, Semm K. Various coagulation techniques tested in a rabbit model. *Endoscopy* 1984; **16**: 47–52.
12 Beisland HO, Stranden E. Rectal temperature monitoring during Neodymium-YAG laser irradiation for prostatic carcinoma. *Urol Res* 1984; **12**: 257–259.
13 Ramsay JWA *et al*. A comparison of bipolar and monopolar diathermy probes in experimental animals. *Urol Res* 1985; **13**: 99–102.
14 Wagner JW, Phillips LC. Reducing variations in power output measurements of electrosurgical devices. *Med Instr* 1980; **14**: 264.
15 Maudsley RF, Qizilbash AH. Thermal injury to the bowel as a complication of laparoscopic sterilization. *Can J Surg* 1979; **22**: 232–234.
16 Thompson BH, Wheeless CR. Gastrointestinal complications of laparoscopic sterilization. *Obstet Gynaecol* 1973; **41**: 669.
17 Loffer FD, Pent D. Indications, contraindications and complications of laparoscopy. *Obstet Gynaecol Survey* 1975; **30**: 407.
18 Wheeless CR. Gastrointestinal injuries associated with laparoscopy. In: Phillips JM (ed) *Endoscopy in Gynaecology*. Downey, California, 1978: 317–324.
19 Peterson HB, Dry H, Greenspan J, Tyler C. Deaths associated with laparoscopic sterilization by unipolar electrocoagulating devices, 1978 and 1979. *Am J Obstet Gynaecol* 1981; **139**: 141.
20 Levy BS, Soderstrom RM, Dail DH. Bowel injuries during laparoscopy: gross anatomy and histology. *J Reprod Med* 1985; **30**: 168.
21 Piercy JRA, Auth DC, Silverstein FE, Willard HR *et al*. Electrosurgical treatment of experimental bleeding canine gastric ulcers. *Gastroenterology* 1978; **74**: 527–534.

22 DiGiovanni M, Vasilenko P, Belski D. Laparoscopic tubal sterilization. The potential for thermal bowel injury. *J Reprod Med* 1990; **35**: 951–954.

23 Voyles CR, Tucker RD. Education and engineering solutions for potential problems with laparoscopic monopolar electrosurgery. *Am J Surg* 1992; **164**: 57–62.

24 Hunter JG. Laser or electrocautery for laparoscopic cholecystectomy? *Am J Surg* 1991; **161**: 345–349.

25 Way LW. Bile duct injury during laparoscopic cholecystectomy. *Ann Surg* 1992; **215**: 195 (Editorial).

26 Ragins H, Shinya H, Wolff WI. The explosive potential of caloric gas during colonoscopic polypectomy. *Surg Gynecol Obstet* 1974; **138**: 554.

27 Bigard MA, Gaucher P, Lasalle C. Fatal colonic explosion during colonoscopic polypectomy. *Gastroenterology* 1979; **77**: 1307–1310.

28 Branday JM. Jejunal gas explosion resulting from the use of diathermy. *Br J Surg* 1982; **69**: 728.

29 Vellar DJ, Pucius R, Vellar ID. Explosion injury of the proximal jejunum caused by diathermy in a patient with obstructing sclerosing peritonitis. *Br J Surg* 1986; **73**: 157–158.

30 Rioux JE. Relative risks of unipolar versus bipolar electrocoagulation. In: Phillips JM (ed.) *Endoscopy in Gynaecology*. Downey, California, 1978: 312–315.

31 LoCicero J, Quebbeman EJ, Nichols RL. Health hazards in the operating room. *Bull Am Coll Surgeons* 1987; **72**: 4–9.

32 Levine RL, Reich H. Advances in gynecologic laparoscopy. *World J Surgery* 1993; **17**: 63–69.

33 Baumann H, Jaeger P, Huch A. Ureteral injury after laparoscopic tubal sterilisation by bipolar electrocoagulation. *Obstet Gynecol* 1988; **71**: 483–485.

34 Strasberg SM, Sanabria JR, Clavien PA. Complications of laparoscopic cholecystectomy. *Can J Surg* 1992; **35**: 275–280.

35 The Southern Surgeons Club. A prospective analysis of 1518 laparoscopic cholecystectomies. *N Engl J Med* 1991; **324**: 1073–1078.

36 Litwin DEM, Girotti MJ, Poulin EC, Mamazza J, Nagy AG *et al.* Laparoscopic cholecystectomy: Trans-Canada experience with 2201 cases. *Can J Surg* 1992; **35**: 291–296.

37 Leahy AL, Bouchier-Hayes DB, Hyland JM, Delaney PV, O'Sullivan G, Keane FB *et al.* Early experiences of laparoscopic cholecystectomy in five Irish hospitals. *Irish J Med Sci* 1992; **161**(60): 410–413.

38 Perissat J. Laparoscopic cholecystectomy: gateway to the future. *Am J Surg* 1991; **161**: 408 (Editorial).

39 Monson JRT, Darzi A, Carey PD, Guillou PJ. Prospective evaluation of laparoscopic-assisted colectomy in an unselected group of patients. *Lancet* 1992; **340**: 831–833.

40 Cortesi N, Ferrari P, Zumbarda E *et al.* Diagnosis of bilateral abdominal cryptorchidism by laparoscopy. *Endoscopy* 1976; **8**: 33.

41 Winfield HN, Donovan JF, See WA, Loening SA, Williams RD. Urological laparoscopic surgery. *J Urol* 1991; **146**: 941–948.

42 Ferguson CM. Electrosurgical laparoscopic cholecystectomy. *Am Surg* 1992; **58**: 96–99.

43 Voyles CR, Petro AB, Meena AL, Haick AJ, Koury AM. A practical approach to laparoscopic cholecystectomy. *Am J Surg* 1991; **161**: 365–370.

44 Hurst BS, Awoniyi CA, Stephens JK *et al.* Application of the cavitron ultrasonic surgical aspirator (CUSA) for laparoscopic surgery using the rabbit as an animal model. *Fertil Steril* 1992; **58**: 444–448.

45 Hodgeson WJ, Delguercio LR. Preliminary experience in liver surgery using the ultrasonic scalpel. *Surgery* 1984; **95**: 230–234.

46 Cuschieri A, Berci G (eds) Instruments and basic techniques for laparoscopic surgery. In: *Laparoscopic Biliary Surgery*, 2nd edn. Blackwell Scientific Publications, Oxford, 1992: 26–68.

47 Wetter LA, Payne JH, Kirshenbaum G, Podoll EF. The ultrasonic dissector facilitates laparoscopic cholecystectomy. *Arch Surg* 1992; **127**: 1195–1198.

Chapter 15

Endoscopic guided surface repair of inguinal hernia: mini hernia repair

A. Darzi and C. Nduka

The surgical approach to inguinal hernias continues to undergo technical modifications. Traditional repairs of McVay, Bassini and Shouldice are achieved by the union of non-anatomically opposed tissues under tension [1–3]. These operation often result in lengthy, painful recovery periods and have reported recurrence rates ranging from 3 to 21% for a primary repair [4–8]. Laparoscopic hernia repair as described by Ger [9, 10] has shown short-term advantages over traditional approaches in terms of postoperative pain and return to work. However, the operation is technically demanding and the long-term results are unknown. With recurrence rates of only 0.7% [11], Lichtenstein's 'tension-free hernioplasty' using a prosthetic mesh should be the standard against which new hernia repairs are measured. We describe a novel tension-free repair, the mini-herniorrhaphy, performed through a 2 cm incision with the aid of laparoscopic instrumentation.

Patients and methods

Between October 1993 and January 1994, one of the authors (A.D.) performed mini-herniorrhaphy on 52 patients. Fifty patients had unilateral primary hernias, and two patients had bilateral hernias. The mean age was 49 years (range 19–69 years). There were 51 males and one female.

Surgical technique

The procedure is performed under general anaesthesia. The patient is placed in a supine position and draped as for an open hernia repair. A 2 cm incision is made in the skin at the level of the internal inguinal ring (Fig. 15.1). The subcutaneous tissues are bluntly dissected down to the external oblique aponeurosis and a 1 cm incision made in it parallel to its fibres (Fig. 15.2). An index finger is inserted into the inguinal canal to separate the external oblique aponeurosis from the spermatic cord down to the level of the external inguinal ring (Fig. 15.3). The finger is withdrawn and a 10 mm laparoscopic fan retractor (Laparofan™, Origin Medsystems Inc, USA) is inserted into the inguinal canal under direct vision (Fig. 15.4). The retractor blades

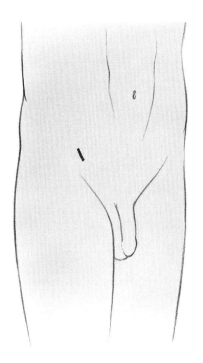

Figure 15.1
A 2 cm incision at the internal ring.

are spread and locked into an open position and the device attached to the abdominal wall lift (Laparolift™, Origin Medsystems Inc, USA). The arm is raised, thus retracting the abdominal wall and creating a working space in the inguinal canal. A 5 mm laparoscope, connected to routine video-imaging equipment, is inserted into the inguinal canal (Fig. 15.5). This arrangement allows the inguinal canal to be visualized directly using light from the laparoscope, and also allows a magnified image of the canal to be viewed on the television monitor.

Endoscopic short grasping and dissecting instruments (Endo-shears, Endo Dissect Short, AutoSuture, UK) are inserted into the canal and the spermatic cord mobilized from the floor of the inguinal canal (Fig. 15.6). The spermatic cord is grasped and a

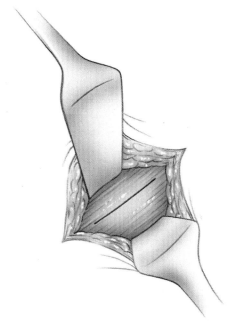

Figure 15.2
The subcutaneous tissue is bluntly dissected to the external oblique aponeurosis and a 2 cm incision is made through the external oblique.

Figure 15.3
An index finger is inserted into the canal mobilizing the cord off the undersurface of the external oblique aponeurosis.

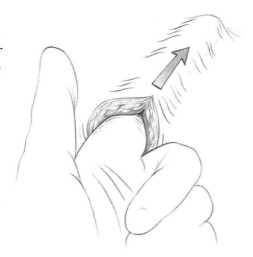

'window' is created between the spermatic cord and the floor of the inguinal canal near the pubic tubercle. A tape is passed around the spermatic cord using curved conventional instruments. When elevating the spermatic cord, great care should be taken to include the external spermatic vessels and the ilioinguinal nerve with the cord. This ensures that the genital nerve is preserved.

Following mobilization of the cord from the floor of the inguinal canal, the laparoscopic fan retractor is removed and the spermatic cord delivered through the skin incision by pulling the two ends of the tape (Fig. 15.7). An incision is made in the spermatic cord and its contents are inspected for the presence of a hernial sac. Where a sac is identified it is mobilized, divided, and the peritoneal end sutured (Fig. 15.8). The laparoscopic fan retractor is then reinserted and placed below the spermatic cord and the external oblique aponeurosis. The retractor is once again raised thus providing good exposure of the inguinal canal.

A sheet of monofilament polypropylene mesh measuring 8×13 cm is fashioned (AutoSuture Company, Ascot, UK). If necessary this may be trimmed by 1–2 cm to match the varying sizes of the inguinal floor. The mesh is inserted into the inguinal

Figure 15.4
The Laparofan is inserted into the inguinal canal under direct vision.

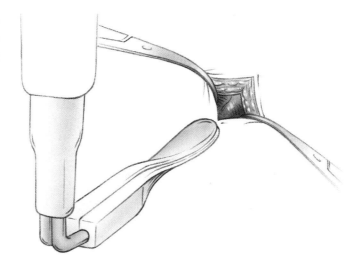

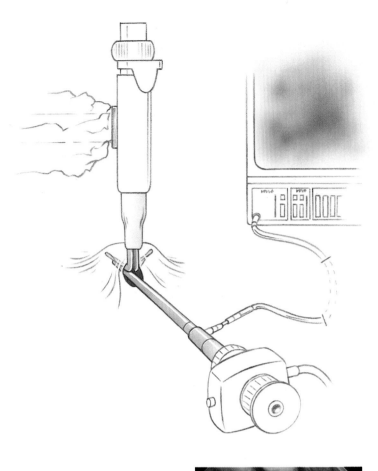

Figure 15.5
The abdominal wall and the roof of the inguinal canal are elevated, creating space within the inguinal canal for the introduction of a 5 mm video-endoscope.

canal under laparoscopic guidence using two anchoring sutures (Fig. 15.9). The mesh is then anchored medially to the rectus sheath, the internal oblique aponeurosis or muscle above and to the inguinal ligament below, using an automatic stapling device (Versatack^{TM}, AutoSuture UK) (Fig. 15.10). A slit in the mesh at the internal ring allows emergence of the spermatic cord and creates two tails. The tails of the mesh are crossed over without tension, wrapped around the cord and stapled to Poupart's ligament lateral to the inguinal ring. When the retractor is released the mesh should buckle slightly. This laxity is desirable to ensure a true tension-free repair and is taken up when the patient strains postoperatively.

The external oblique aponeurosis is closed over the cord using a single absorbable chromic catgut suture. The wound is sprayed with antiseptic solution and the skin closed with steri strips (Fig. 15.11). Patients are discharged within 24 h of the operation with minimal postoperative pain for which mild analgesics are prescribed. Unrestricted activity is encouraged.

Figure 15.6
The spermatic cord is mobilized using endoscopic graspers.

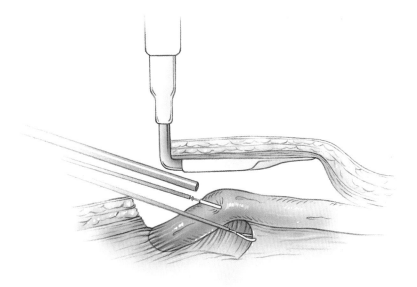

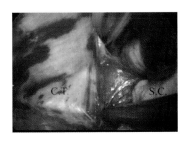

Figure 15.7
The spermatic cord is delivered through the incision and an incision is made along its anterior surface to identify the indirect inguinal sac.

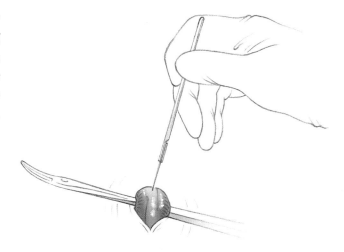

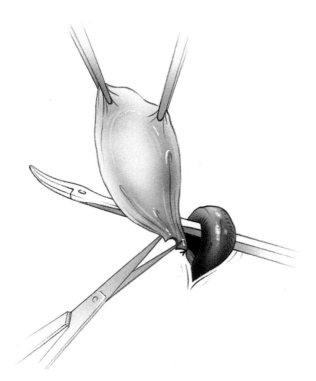

Figure 15.8
An indirect inguinal sac identified and mobilized off the cord and divided.

Results

The mean operative time was 45 min (range 25–74 min). In 28 out of 54 cases the hernia was indirect. All of the patients left hospital on the day following surgery and resumed normal activity within 2–10 days. The complications to date include scrotal swelling (*n*=1), urinary retention (*n*=1) and serous wound discharge (*n*=1) (follow-up period 0–3 months).

Discussion

The role of laparoscopic herniorrhaphy is currently a matter of much debate [12–17] (see also Chapter 6). Less pain, no muscle incision, a tension-free repair and an earlier return to work have all been quoted as advantages of minimally invasive surgery over more traditional approaches. However, as the laparoscopic repair necessitates violation of the peritoneal cavity, it is debatable whether it really does represent a less-invasive procedure. The operation is potentially fraught with a number of complications resulting from its trans-abdominal approach [18]. These may include injuries to the bladder, nerves or blood vessels resulting from an inappropriate application of diathermy, staples or sutures. There is also the possibility of bowel obstruction resulting from the formation of adhesions at the site of peritoneal closure [19]. Laparoscopic herniorrhaphy is a minimal access procedure, not a minimally invasive one. Successful completion of the operation thus requires a detailed understanding of inguinal anatomy as viewed from inside the peritoneal cavity [17], not to mention considerable hand–instrument–eye coordination. Laparoscopic extraperitoneal hernia repair has been advocated to avoid some of the pitfalls of a transabdominal approach [20, 21], but this is an even more technically demanding procedure.

Figure 15.9
The mesh is inserted into the inguinal canal using anchoring sutures.

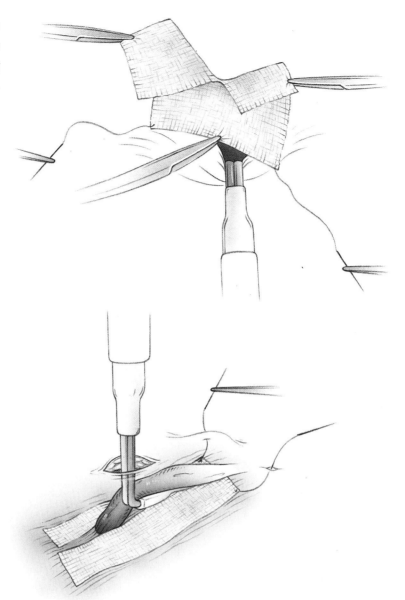

Lichtenstein's tension-free repair has several advantages over laparoscopic approaches. The most important of these are that the repair can be performed under local anaesthetic using a familiar anatomical approach without violating the peritoneal cavity. However, although the operation has shown its long-term safety and effectiveness, it still requires a skin incision of up to 8–10 cm.

The mini-herniorrhaphy described above maintains all of the advantages of the tension-free repair whilst adding the benefits of a minimally invasive procedure. Specifically, it is achieved through a much smaller incision (on average 2 cm or less) than any previous repair, yet through the use of an endoscope provides a magnified view of the operative field. Furthermore, the external oblique aponeurosis is not fully divided as with the Lichtenstein repair; all that is required is a 1–2 cm incision to allow access to the inguinal canal. The procedure also allows operation under direct vision by using the endoscope as a light source. Thus, in contrast to laparoscopy, the operation

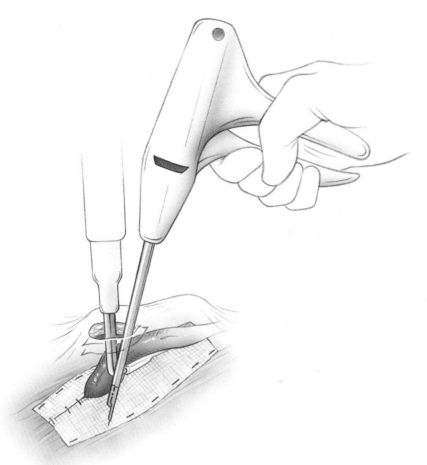

Figure 15.10
The mesh is stapled to the inguinal ligament using the Versatak stapler.

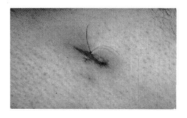

Figure 15.11
Incision closed.

is carried out under stereoscopic vision whilst maintaining the important sensory cues of touch and feel. Any problems resulting from visualizing unfamiliar, endoscopically viewed anatomy are eliminated as the operation is carried out using a familiar approach. In addition, the use of the stapler allows the mesh to be rapidly anchored in place without the need for sutures, which would require a larger skin incision. Whilst being perfected, we have performed the mini-herniorrhaphy using a general anaesthetic. However, the operation may also be performed under local anaesthetic.

During early development of the mini-herniorrhaphy, retraction of the abdominal wall was achieved with the aid of a pharyngoscope through which was inserted the 5 mm endoscope. However, considerable manual traction was needed to gain adequate exposure of the inguinal canal. We therefore employed the laparoscopic fan retractor attached to a mechanical abdominal wall lift. These devices have increasingly been used as an alternative to carbon dioxide insufflation during laparoscopy, particularly on patients with ventilatory difficulties [22, 23]. In mini-hernia repair the laparoscopic fan retractor allows better exposure of the inguinal canal and thus easier positioning of the mesh.

Finally, of course, there is the issue of cost. This approach almost totally avoids the use of large numbers of expensive disposable laparoscopic instruments. The use of the open stapling device as described is, however, considered necessary to facilitate fixation of the mesh through such restricted access.

This is the first description of a surface approach to inguinal hernia repair that combines the virtues of a tension-free repair with minimal tissue trauma and reduced wound size. The important traditional surgical principles of 3-D vision and full tactile feedback are maintained, therefore allowing the margins of the defect to be both seen and felt. We have had no recurrences to date, but our follow-up period is obviously too short to allow any definite conclusions to be drawn. However, there is no reason to expect our recurrence rate to be any higher than that of Lichtenstein (less than 1%). The follow-up times of any large series of laparoscopic herniorrhaphies are too short to make a direct comparison with the tension-free repair. Nevertheless, we envisage that the mini-herniorrhaphy may signify the premature demise of laparoscopic repair for a primary inguinal hernia.

References

1 McVay CB. Inguinal and femoral hernioplasty: anatomical repair. *Arch Surg* 1948; **57**: 524.
2 Bassini E. Spora 100 casi di cura radicali dell'ernia inguinale operata col. methodo dell'autore. *Arch Atti Soc Ital Chir* 1888; **5**: 315.
3 Shouldice EE. The treatment of hernia. *Ontario Med Rev* 1953; 1–4.
4 Wantz GE. Shouldice repair. *Cont Surg* 1988; **33**: 15–21.
5 Sisley JF, Scarbourough CS, Morris RC *et al.* Shouldice hernia repair: results of a teaching institution. *Am Surg* 1987; **53**: 495-496.
6 Cahlin E, Weiss L. Results of postoperative clinical examination of inguinal hernia after three years. *Acta Chir Scand* 1980; **146**: 421.
7 Asmussen T, Jensen FV. A follow-up study on recurrence after inguinal hernia repair. *Surg Gynecol Obstet* 1983; **156**: 198.
8 Ingimersson O, Spak I. Inguinal and femoral hernias: Long term results in a community hospital. *Acta Chir Scand* 1983; **149**: 291.
9 Ger R, Monroe K, Duvivier R *et al.* Management of indirect inguinal hernias by laparoscopic closure of the neck of the sac. *Am J Surg* 1990; **159**: 320–323.
10 Ger R. The laparoscopic management of groin hernias. *Cont Surg* 1991; **39**: 15–19.
11 Lichtenstein IL. Herniorrhaphy: A personal experience with 6321 cases. *Am J Surg* 1987; **153**: 553–559.
12 Popp L. Transcutaneous aquadissection of the musculofascial defect and pre-peritoneal endoscopic patch repair. *J Laparoendosc Surg* 1991; **1**: 83–90.
13 Schultz L. Laser laparoscopic herniorrhaphy: a clinical trial. *J. Laparoendosc Surg* 1990; **1**: 41–45.
14 Corbitt JD Jr. Laparoscopic herniorrhaphy. *Surg Laparosc Endosc* 1991; **1**: 23–25.
15 Dion Y-M, Morin J. Laparoscopic inguinal herniorrhaphy. *Can J Surg* 1992; **35**: 209–212.
16 Sailors DM, Layman TS, Burns RP, Chandler KE, Russell WL. Laparoscopic hernia repair: a preliminary report. *Am Surg* 1993; **59**: 85–89.
17 Ger R, Mishrick A, Hurwitz J, Romero C, Oddsen R. Management of groin hernias by laparoscopy. *World J Surg* 1993; **17**: 46–50.
18 MacFadyen BV Jr, Arregui ME, Corbitt JD Jr *et al.* Complications of laparoscopic inguinal hernia repair. *Surg Endosc* 1993; **7**: 155–158.
19 Arregui ME, Navarrete J, Davis CJ, Castro D, Nagan RF. Laparoscopic inguinal herniorrhaphy: techniques and controversies. *Surg Clin North Am* 1993; **73**: 513–527.

20 Ferzli GS, Massad A, Albert P. Extraperitoneal endoscopic inguinal hernia repair. *J Laparoendosc Surg* 1992; **2**: 281–286.

21 McKernan JB, Lewis HL. Laparoscopic repair of inguinal hernias using a totally extraperitoneal prosthetic approach. *Surg Endosc* 1993; **7**: 26–28.

22 Hashimoto D, Nayeem SA, Kajiwara S, Hoshino T. Laparoscopic cholecystectomy: an approach without pneumoperitoneum. *Surg Endosc* 1993; **7**: 54–56.

23 Holzman M, Sharp K, Richard W. Hypercarbia during carbon dioxide insufflation for therapeutic laparoscopy: a note of caution. *Surg Laparosc Endosc* 1992; **2**: 11–14.

Acknowledgment

The authors and publisher wish to thank Joanna Cameron for the use of original artwork in this chapter.

Index